MICROBIOLOGY MCQs

120+ MOST PROBABLE MCQs

GETTING YOUR DREAM BRANCH IS NOW EASY

Author

ARHAM FAROOQUI

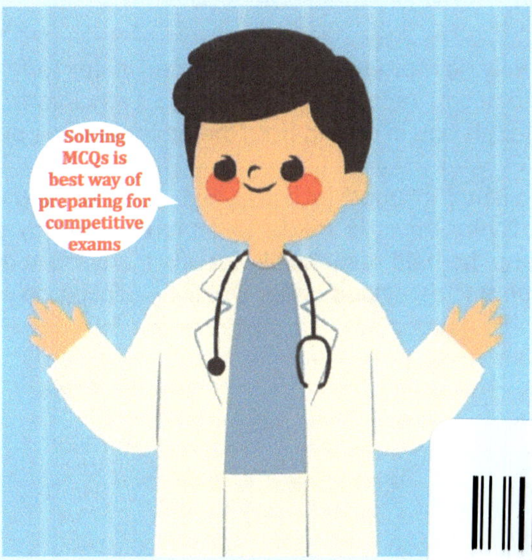

Peepee Publishers and Distributors Private Limited®

MICROBIOLOGY MCQs

Published by
Pawaninder P. Vij and Anupam Vij

Peepee Publishers and Distributors Private Limited
Head Office: 160, Shakti Vihar, Pitam Pura, Delhi-110 034 (India)

Correspondence Address:

7/31, First Floor, Ansari Road, Daryaganj
New Delhi-110 002 (India)

Ph: 41512412, 9811156083

e-mail: peepee160@yahoo.co.in

e-mail: peepee160@gmail.com

www.peepeepub.com

join us on facebook.com/pp.publishers

First Edition: 2024

ISBN: 978-81-9651-875-2

PREFACE

With ever increasing competition in the medical field along with its advances in treatment regimes, it has become fairly common among examiners to assess medical students practical approach and application of their learned knowledge by testing them with clinical scenario-based questions. Acknowledging this shift in paradigm author attempts to prepare and help the students in developing their clinical knowledge, skills and integrating their knowledge of different subjects by solving clinical scenario-based MCQs centered around "Microbiology/Infectious Disease". This book is prepared particularly for medical students preparing for their competitive exams (like NEET–PG/NExT/FMGE/CMSE/USMLE/PLAB/AMC) by providing them 120+ Hypothetical Clinical scenario-based MCQs.

There are almost 100+ images used in this book. The author have been extremely cautious with regards to the copyright and licensing of the images. If there seems to be any query with regards to the licensing or copyright kindly send an email to farooquiarham@yahoo.com. In case of genuine and justified allegation the specified content of the book will be taken down immediately.

Arham Farooqui

CONTENTS

Microbiology MCQs

1. 23 years old male from India presents to general physician with primary complain of fever, fatigue, headache, weakness along with abdominal pain and diarrhea for the last 5 days. On further questioning it was revealed that his fever has followed 'Step ladder patterns' and his diarrhea was most probably 'pea soup diarrhea'.

On physical examination it was found that patient is having 'rose spots' on chest which he denies weren't there earlier. His vitals were stable with no other significant findings.

Based upon symptoms, history and general examination which organism is responsible for patients pathology and what is best selective media to culture this organism?

A. Vibrio cholera; Wilson and Blair brilliant green bismuth sulphite

B. Salmonella typhi; Wilson and Blair brilliant green bismuth sulphite

C. Vibrio cholera; Sorbitol MacConkey agar

D. EHEC; Sorbitol MacConkey agar

Answer: B. Salmonella typhi; Wilson and Blair brilliant green bismuth sulphite

Solution

- This is the case of Typhoid fever or Enteric fever.
- It is caused by certain 'Salmonella'.
- Salmonella typhi (Most common cause in India).
- Salmonella paratyphi A.
- Salmonella paratyphi B.
- Salmonella paratyphi C.
- Rest of Salmonella serotypes are called non-typhoidal Salmonella.
- Salmonella comes under classification of Enterobacteriaceae.
- Based upon 'Kaufmann and White scheme' classification there are over 3000 serotypes of Salmonella. Kaufmann and White scheme is based upon 3 antigens:

  1. H antigen 2. O antigen 3. Vi antigen

Features of these antigen:

1. **H antigen:**

- Flagellar antigen, proteinaceous in nature.
- Heat and alcohol labile in nature.
- Phase variation.
- Highly antigenic.
- Antibodies against H antigen are first to be formed after infection and persist for several months.

2. **O antigen:**
   - It is a somatic antigen, polysaccharide in nature.
   - It is heat and alcohol stable.
   - It has lower antigenicity.
   - Antibodies formed against O antigen appears after H antibodies and disappears by few weeks.
3. **Vi antigen:**
   - It is capsular antigen, polysaccharide in nature.
   - Least antigenic.
   - Heat labile and alcohol stable.
   - Present only in S. typhi, S. paratyphi C.
   - Vi antibody appears for short time during convalescence.

"Persistence of Vi antibody means person is carrier."

Typhoid

- **Etiology:** Generally Typhoid is spread by 'feco-oral' route or 'urine-oral' route.
- Typhoid is contagious in a way that it is present in fecal matter of infected person.
- Typhoid is most often seen in countries or places with poor sanitation where water supply or food gets contaminated by fecal matter.
- **Incubation period:** 3-10 days.
- Typhoid or Enteric fever is caused by 'Salmonella' which is member of Enterobacteriaceae.
- Salmonella is gram-negative rod shaped facultative anaerobe.

Biochemical Properties of Salmonella

1. Catalase positive.
2. Oxidase negative.
3. Voges-Proskauer positive.
4. Methyl red test positive.
5. Urease test negative.
6. Indole test negative.

- On blood agar Salmonella is gamma hemolytic in nature.

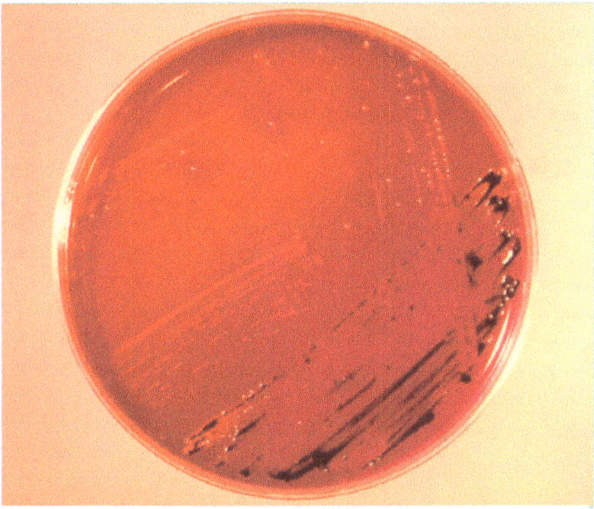

This photograph depicts the colonial growth pattern displayed by the bacterium, Salmonella enterica subsp. arizonae, which had been grown on a medium of xylose lysine deoxycholate (XLD) agar

Clinical Features: Malaise Symptoms:

- Step ladder fever (Faget's sign) is very characteristic and diagnostic feature of Typhoid.
- Also there is diarrhea which is described as pea soup diarrhea.
- There can also be presence of red spots on body.
- Disease is mostly self-limiting and remains for 3-4 weeks.

Diagnosis:

- For first week we take blood sample.
- From second week presence of Salmonella increases in intestine therefore from second week recommend sample is fecal matter.
- From third week recommend sample is urine (although rare cause most patients starts to recover by that time).
- One of the unique test for Typhoid is 'Widal test', it detects presence of H and O antigen.
- Best medium for culture of Salmonella is 'Wilson and Blair' bismuth sulphite agar.
- **Other methods include:**
  1. Microscopy; gram staining.
  2. Serology like ELISA.
  3. Molecular methods like PCR and NAAT's.
- **Treatment:** Drug of choice is Ciprofloxacin.

2. 19 years old female presents to general physician with primary complain of fever, fatigue, headache, weakness along with abdominal pain and bloody diarrhea for the last 2 days. Patient tells that in her locality there have been several instances of people getting ill due to poor sanitary. Based on this consulting doctor conducted Wet mount test for his stool sample which showed following observations.

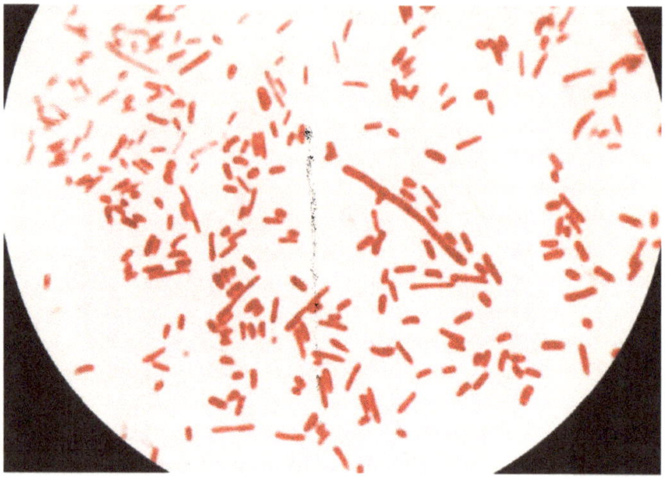

Gram-negative, rod-shaped, Shigella dysenteriae bacteria

Which of the following is NOT correct regarding pathogenic organism?

A. Ciprofloxacin is Drug of Choice

B. Sereny test can be used for diagnosis

C. ELISA for VMA can be used for diagnosis

D. Complications like intussusception, megacolon and HUS can be used for diagnosis

E. Receptor for Shiga toxin is Gb3 present at Endothelial cell of small intestine and kidney

F. It mostly infiltrate duodenum and jejunum

Answer: F. It mostly infiltrate duodenum and jejunum

Solution

- This is the case of bacillary dysentery caused by shigella.
- Shigella comes under classification of Enterobacteriaceae.
- Shigellae are gram-negative, nonmotile, facultatively anaerobic, non-spore-forming rods.
- **Mode of Infection:** Feco-oral route.
- **Clinical Features:** Abdominal pain, diarrhea, dysentery.
- **Complications:** Toxic megacolon, intussusception, Hemolytic Uremic Syndrome.

Diagnosis:

1. **Gram smear:** Salmonella along with pus and RBC in stool.
2. Serological methods like ELISA.
3. Sereny test.
4. Invasion of Hela/Help-2 cell line.

Drug of Choice: Ciprofloxacin.

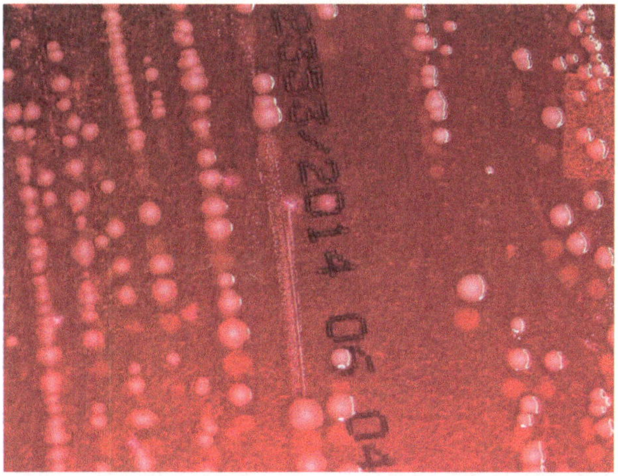

Under the low-power, 10X magnification of a digital keyence scope, this figure depicts the colonial growth displayed by gram-negative, Shigella sonnei bacteria, which were cultured on xylose-lysine-deoxycholate (XLD) agar medium, for a 48-hour time period, at a temperature of 37°C

List of Lactose and Non-Lactose Fermenting Enterobacteriaceae

- *Lactose fermenting (Mnemonic—CEEK)*
  1. Citrobacter
  2. Enterobacter
  3. Klebsiella
  4. E. coli
- *Non-Lactose fermenting bacteria*
  P 1. Proteus
  S 2. Shigella
  M 3. Morgnella
  P 4. Providencia
  S 5. Salmonella
  Y 6. Yersinia
- Lactose fermenting bacteria on MacConkey medium manifest as 'pink' color.
- While non-lactose fermenting bacteria on MacConkey medium manifest as 'pale' color.

3. 35 years old male comes to an ER with severe flank pain and pain in genital. Pain was severe in intensity sharp and consistent in nature. According to Numeric Pain Scale Intensity of pain was 8/10. Attendee along with patient tells that for the last 2 weeks patient is having increased frequency and urgency for urination. Patient is heavy smoker consumed 1 pack every day for the last 15 years. Patient had ischemic stroke 2 months back for which he underwent surgery. Patient has history of uncontrolled hypertension, dyslipidemia along with diabetes mellitus type 2. On physical examination patient vitals were as follows – pulse rate of 92, blood pressure of 188/98 and respiratory rate was 22. Based on this what is the diagnosis for patients current pain and what is the cause for it?

A. Acute Hemolytic Transfusion Reaction; caused by ABO incompatibility in blood transfusion

B. Renal stones; caused by Proteus

C. Renal stones; caused by E. coli

D. Acute Kidney Injury; Post operative complication

Answer: B. Renal stones; caused by Proteus

Solution

- In the given question Option A is not possible because Acute Blood Transfusion Reaction occurs within 24 hours of blood transfusion and patient underwent surgery 2 months ago.
- Since patient underwent surgery 2 months ago hence option D, i.e., post operative AKI is not possible.
- As it is given patient is having increased frequency and urgency for urination indicating towards Urinary Tract Infection and the most common UTI forming renal stone and causing flank pain and referred genital pain is 'Proteus'. Also since it is given in question that patient had ischemic stroke which must have been followed by long-term catheterization which is most common mode of transmission for Proteus.

Proteus

- It comes under classification of Enterobacteriaceae.
- It is gram-negative, motile and non-capsulated.

Biochemical Reactions:

- Produces Hydrogen disulfide gas on sugar fermentation.
- PPA test positive (converts phenylalanine into phenyle pyruvic acid by producing deaminase enzyme).
- On MacConkey medium-Non lactose fermenting with very characteristic fishy smell.
- On blood agar it exhibit swarming (Diene's phenomenon).
- IMViC:++--(Indole positive, Methyl red positive, Voges-Proskauer test negative, Citrate test negative.
- Urease positive means converts urea to ammonia and carbon dioxide.
- This urease enzyme is responsible for increasing urine pH turning it to basic which is responsible for renal stone formation.
- Proteus is responsible for formation of triphosphate or staghorn or struvite stone.
- Most common Mode of transmission of Proteus is long-term use of catheterization, generally seen after ischemic or hemorrhagic stroke or liver transplant surgery.
- Types of infection it causes:
  1. Wound infection.
  2. Intraabdominal abscess.
  3. Peritonitis.
  4. Nasocomial pneumonia.
- **Drug of Choice for Proteus:** Aminoglycosides and cephalosporins.

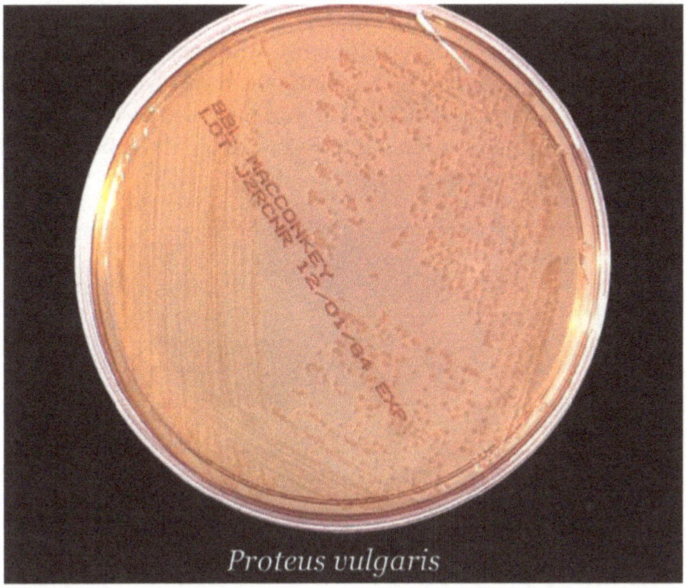

After 24 hours, this inoculated MacConkey agar culture plate cultivated colonial growth of gram-negative, rod-shaped and facultatively anaerobic, Proteus vulgaris bacteria

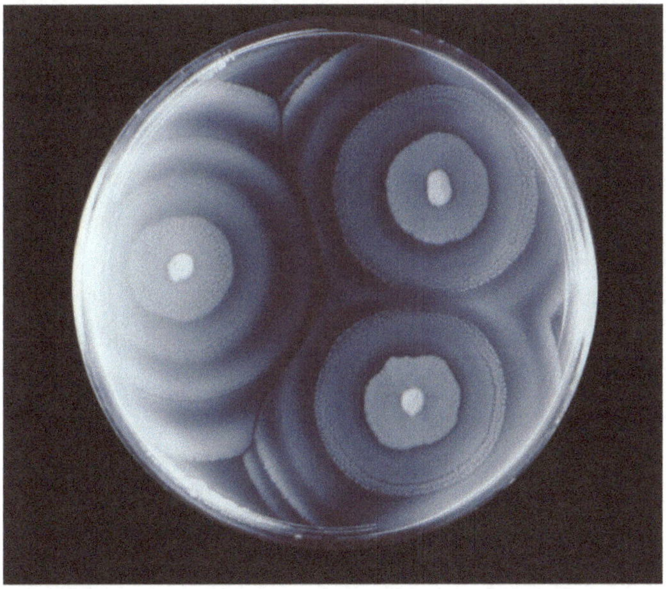

This figure depicts a Petri dish culture plate, which had contained a trypticase soy agar growth medium, that had been inoculated with Proteus mirabilis bacteria and subsequently gave rise to this colonial growth pattern referred to the Dienes reaction

4. 17 years old male comes to physician with complain of abdominal pain and bloody diarrhea for the last 4 days. There is no associated history of nausea or vomiting. There is no associated recent travel history and patient says that he has mainly remained on his usual dietary pattern. On physical examination there are no lesions present and his vitals were stable. Patient was asked to undergo blood culture which revealed presence of E. coli as given below in the image. Which of the following E. coli is responsible for patient's condition?

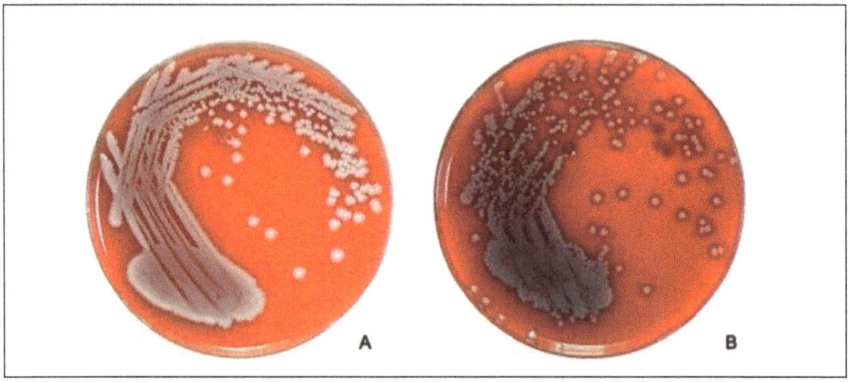

Most strains of E. coli produce smooth, circular, low-convex colonies with entire edge that are about 3-4 mm in diameter. They are greyish, butyrous and readily emulsified

Source: Wikipedia; Author: Hans N; License: Creative Commons Attribution-ShareAlike 4.0 International license

A. Enteroaggregative E. coli (EAEC)
B. Enterohemorrhagic E. coli (EHEC)
C. Enteropathogenic E. coli (EPEC)
D. Enterotoxigenic E. coli (ETEC)

Answer: B. Enterohemorrhagic E. coli (EHEC)

Solution

- E. coli comes under classification of Enterobacteriaceae.
- **General Biochemical Characteristics of E. coli.:**
  1. Urease test negative (i.e., don't convert urea into ammonia and carbon dioxide.
  2. Do not produce hydrogen di sulphide on sugar fermentation.
  3. IMViC:++--(Indole test positive, methyl red positive, Voges Proskauer negative, Citrate negative.
  4. MacConkey medium–Lactose fermenting.
  5. Blood agar–beta hemolytic.
- E. coli are divided into serotypes on the basis of–O antigen, K antigen, H antigen.
- **E. coli is further classified into 5 types:**
  1. Enterohemorrhagic E. coli (EHEC).
  2. Enteropathogenic E. coli (EPEC).
  3. Enterotoxigenic E. coli (ETEC).
  4. Enteroinvasive E. coli (EIEC).
  5. Enteroaggregative E. coli (EAEC).

- The only E. coli which cause bloody diarrhea is Enterohemorrhagic E. coli.

Enterohemorrhagic E. coli:

- Reservoir–found in GI of cow (zoonoses).
- Most common food to get infection from Beef/Hamburger, contaminated salad, contaminated water, fomites.

Clinical Features:

- Fever, fatigue, bloody diarrhea (very characteristic).
- It is most common cause for Hemolytic Uremic Syndrome HUS (Generally caused by E. coli O157:H7 serotype).
- **Incubation Period:** 3-8 days.

Mechanism of Action/Toxins:

- Locus of enterocyte effacement plasmid: A-E effect.There is attachment to cup-like pedestal with effacement villi.
- Phage mediated Shiga like toxin or verocytotoxin.

Diagnosis:

- Gram smear (specimen–Stool).
- Culture for E. coli–Sorbitol Mac test.
- Sorbitol Mac test give 'pale color' for O157:H7.
- While for rest of E. coli it gives 'pink color'.
- While for non O157:H7 EHEC cytotoxicity on vero cell line is done.

PATHOGENS RESPONSIBLE FOR BLOODY DIARRHEA OR DYSENTERY

B Bacillus.
Y Yersenia.
S Salmonella, Shigella, Schistosoma intercalatum.
E E. coli [EHEC(E. coli O157:H7) and EPEC (Certain strains only)].
E Entamoeba histolytica (Parasite).
C Campylobacter, Clostridium perfringens.

- Mnemonic used is "BY SEC".
- Except for Entamoeba histolytica, Schistosoma intercalatum all are bacteria.
- Schistosoma intercalatum is known to cause Katayama fever.

5. 17 years old male comes to physician with complain of abdominal pain and bloody diarrhea for the last 4 days. Patient was asked to undergo blood culture and sorbitol Mac test resulting in diagnosis of EHEC O157:H7. What treatment should be given to this patient?

A. Ceftriaxone
B. Ampicillin
C. Symptomatic treatment
D. Ciprofloxacin

Answer: C. Symptomatic treatment

Solution

- Since patient is diagnosed with EHEC therefore only symptomatic treatment should be given because antibodies are contraindicated in EHEC cause it increases the risk of HUS (Hemolytic Uremic Syndrome).

6. **21 years old female presents with complain of mild fever, fatigue and diarrhea. Fever was 100.6 °C and diarrhea was non bloody with no mucous. There is no history of recent travel but patient do gives a history of going to local restaurant downtown for dinner 1 day ago. Based on this gram staining for stool specimen was conducted which showed pink colour rod shaped gram-negative bacteria. Then after multiple serologies diagnosis of Enteroinvasive E. coli was made. What would have been finding noticed on stool examination?**

   A. Pus cell positive and RBC's negative along with pink colour gram-negative E. coli
   B. Pus cell negative and RBC's negative with pink colour gram-negative E. coli
   C. Pus cell negative and RBC's negative with pink colour gram-negative E. coli
   D. Pus cell positive and RBC's positive along with pink colour gram-negative E. coli

   Answer: D. Pus cell positive and RBC's positive along with pink colour gram-negative E. coli

Solution

- Mechanism of action for EIEC.
- It produces disease not by toxic substances but invasion which is mediated by plasmid coded antigen called Virulence Marker Antigen (VMA).
- Since it causes invasion so there is presence of RBC's and pus cells.
- Gram smear with pink colour gram-negative E. coli along with RBC's positive and pus cell positive seen in EIEC, EPEC (only certain strains bloody diarrhea), EHEC.
- Gram smear with pink colour gram-negative E. coli with no RBC or pus cell seen in ETEC, EAEC (in some cases EAEC can also cause bloody diarrhea).

7. **30 years old male comes with complain of mild fever, the fatigue and diarrhea for the last 3 days. Fever was 100.8 °C. Diarrhea had no mucous or presence of blood. There was no associated history of nausea or vomiting. Upon conducting gram smear on stool specimen it was found out to be pink colour gram-negative rod shaped organism along with RBC's and pus cell. What are atypical features for this organism?**

   A. Non lactose fermenting
   B. IMViC:++--
   C. Gram-positive
   D. Urease test positive

   Answer: A. Non lactose fermenting

Solution

- Based upon gram smear it has to be either EIEC or EHEC. But since patient don't have history of bloody diarrhea therefore it is most likely to be EIEC.

- EIEC or diarrheagenic E. coli is considered to be atypical E. coli because it is non lactose fermenting and non motile unlike other E. coli.

8. 60 years old male underwent coronary bypass surgery after MI 1 week ago and have been on ventilator. Recently his blood oxygen started going down and difficulty in breathing upon further investigating it was patient having pneumonia with no other CVS abnormality. Upon further investigation it was found patient was infected with pseudomonas aeruginosa. Which of the following is NOT correct for this organism?

A. Catalase positive and oxidase positive

B. Monotrichous

C. Non lactose fermenting with fishy smell

D. Can grow at 42°C and grow in moist environment

E. Most common cause for health care associated pneumonia

Answer: C. Non lactose fermenting with fishy smell

Solution

General Characteristics of Pseudomonas:

1. Gram-negative bacilli.
2. Monotrichous.
3. Non capsulated; instead of capsule it produces slime.

Biochemical Reactions for Pseudomonas:

1. Catalase positive and oxidase positive.
2. Nitrate reduction positive (i.e., nitrate reductase enzyme present).
3. Blood agar-beta Hemolytic mucoid colonies.
4. On nutrient agar produces pigments–pyomelanin, pyorubin, pyoverdine, pyocyanin.
5. MacConkey medium–Non lactose fermenting.
6. Selective medium-Cetrimide agar (fruity smell or grape or sweet smelling colonies).

Note: Since cetrimide is also a strong disinfectant and Pseudomonas are able to grow on cetrimide therefore Pseudomonas are resistant to cetrimide disinfectant.

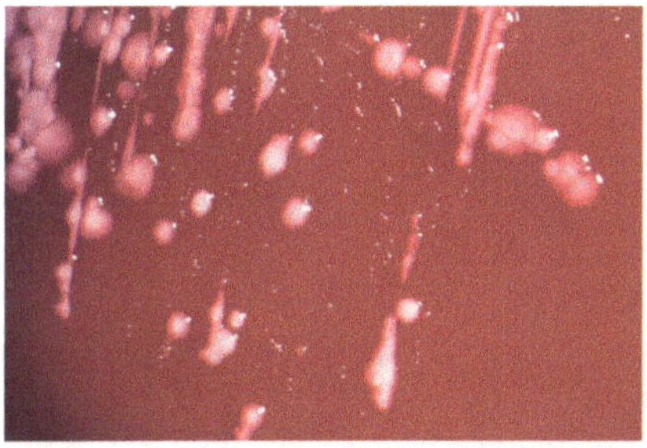

Blood agar-beta hemolytic mucoid colonies seen in Pseudomonas

Content Provider(s): CDC/Dr. Theo Hawkins; License: Creative Commons Attribution-ShareAlike license

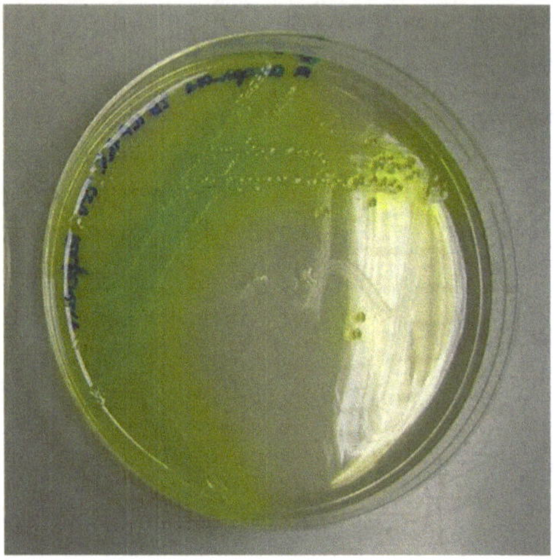

Cetrimide agar with pseudomonas colonies

BACTERIA CAUSING PNEUMONIA

- **PSEUDOMONAS**
- **ACTINOMYCES**
- **STREPTOCOCCUS**
- **CHLAMYDIA**
- **MYCOPLASMA**
- **LEGIONELLA**
- **HAEMOPHILUS INFLUENZA**
- **NOCARDIA**
- **STAPHYLOCOCCUS**
- **KLEBSIELLA**
- **MORAXELLA**

9. 26 years old male comes up with following presentation (as given below in image). Upon taking his history. He told that 4 days back he got severely burned by hot utensil for which he himself did the wound dressing at home. And few days later present with the following presentation (given below in the image).

Which other pathology is NOT caused by the organism responsible for patient's presentation?

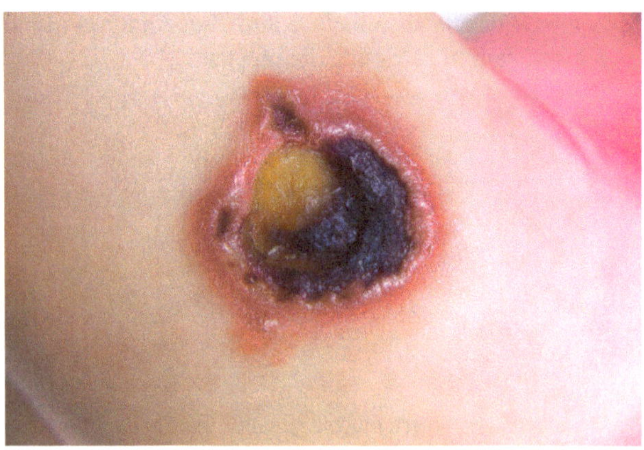

A. Corneal ulcer
B. Simple otitis externa or swimmers ear
C. Shanghai fever
D. Malignant otitis media
E. Hot hand and foot syndrome
F. HUS (Hemolytic Uremic Syndrome)

Answer: F. HUS (Hemolytic Uremic Syndrome)

Solution

- The presentation given in the image is that of Ecthyma gangrenosum which is caused by Pseudomonas aeruginosa.
- Pseudomonas aeruginosa is generally found in moist environment and is known to cause following pathologies:
  1. Corneal ulcer.
  2. Simple otitis media/swimmers ear, can also cause malignant otitis in diabetic and immunosuppressants.
  3. Green nail syndrome.
  4. Hot hand foot syndrome.
  5. Shanghai fever.
  6. Jacuzi/hot tub folliculitis.
  7. Most common cause of burn infection.
  8. Most common cause for ventilator associated pneumonia.
  9. Most common cause for health care associated pneumonia.

10. 28 years old male who is car washer comes with the following presentation as given below. What is the cause for patient's condition?

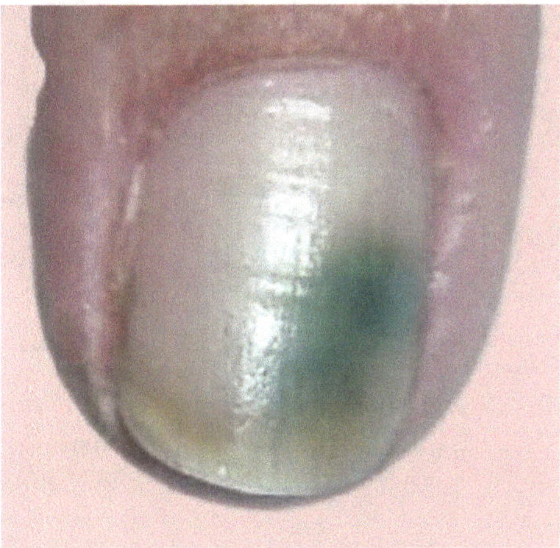

A. Pseudomonas aeruginosa
B. Candida
C. Dermatophytes
D. Rheumatic cause

Answer: A. Pseudomonas aeruginosa

Solution

- The condition shown in above image is that of Green nail syndrome which is caused by Pseudomonas aeruginosa. This is seen with individual who are in constant contact of water like in profession of washing utensils or car wash etc.
- Pseudomonas aeruginosa is also known to cause Jacuzzi/hot tub folliculitis and hot hand/foot syndrome.

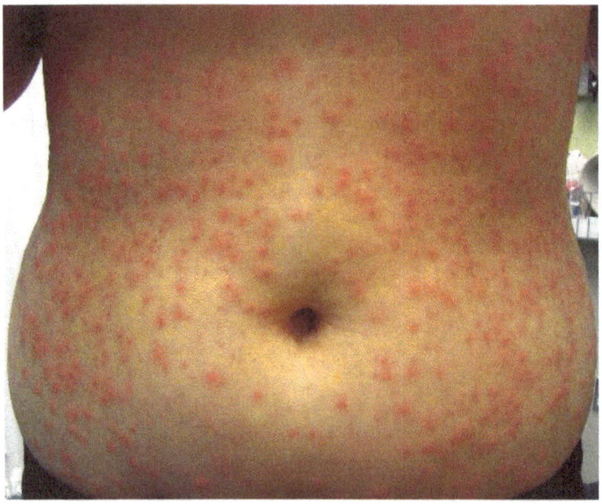

Hot tub folliculitis generally seen in individual who swim in water infected by Pseudomonas aeruginosa

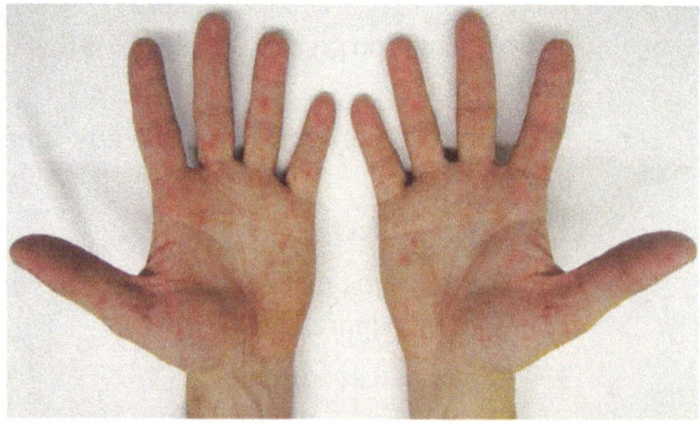

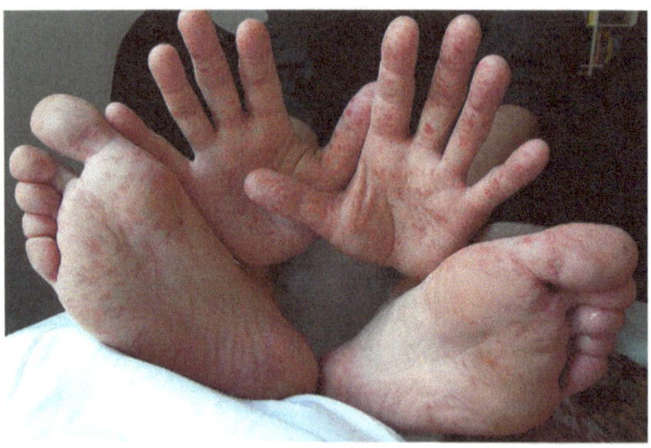

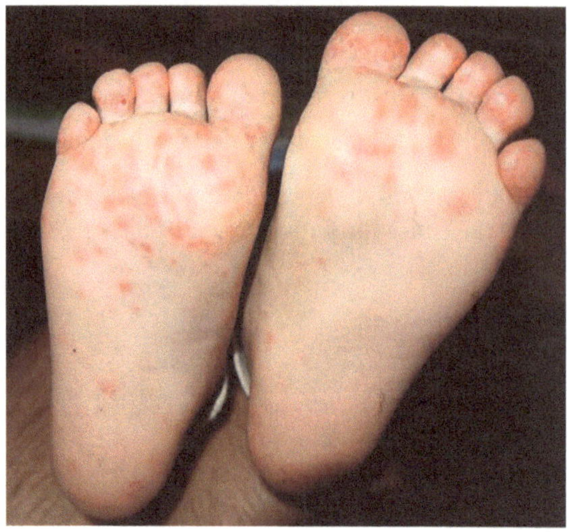

Hot hand and foot syndrome generally occurs when swimmer touches the floor of the pool inhabited by Pseudomonas aeruginosa

11. 36 years old male comes with complain of abdominal pain and watery diarrhea for 3 days. Pain was continuous and cramping in nature and his bowel movement were 3-4 times a day. He has a travel history of travelling to North India. He is non alcoholic, non smoker with no history of drug abuse. Upon performing gram smear and other biochemical test it was to be gram-negative pink colour rod shaped bacteria with no RBC's or pus cell, along with that it was found to be fermenting lactose on MacConkey medium, IMViC:++--, Beta Hemolytic on blood agar. Based on this diagnosis of ETEC was made. What toxins are involved in pathogenicity of ETEC?

A. VMA Virulence Marker Antigen
B. Heat labile toxin
C. Cholera toxin
D. Enterotoxin

Answer: B. Heat labile toxin

Solution

- ETEC is known to cause Travelers diarrhea. It is commonly transmitted by consumption of contaminated food in Asian, African, Latin American countries.
- ETEC produces both heat labile and heat stable toxins which increases cAMP and cGMP respectively which in turn results in secretion of ion causing diarrhea.
- Also ETEC have colonization factor antigen: Fimbriae and outer membrane protein–helps in adhesion to small intestine mucosa, e,g., CFA1, CFA3, CS1, CS2.

12. 43 years old female underwent BM transplant due to AML. 4 hours later of transplant patient's fever starts to rise slightly. Upon doing proper blood investigation it was found that organism responsible for patients rise in temperature is gram-positive cell in chain or pair along with Catalase negative, Oxidase negative.

Also following test given below in image was found to be positive. Name the most probable organism causing increase in temperature and name of the test shown below.

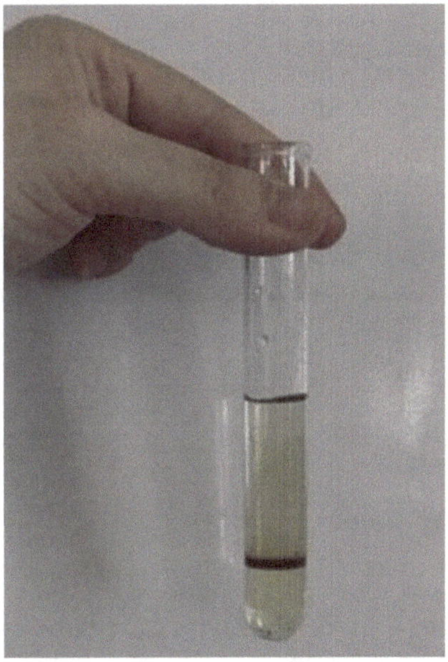

A. Staphylococcus aureus; Coagulase test
B. Streptococcus viridans; Ring precipitation test
C. Bacillus; Gelatin stab test
D. Corynebacterium; Schick

Answer: B. Streptococcus viridans; Ring precipitation test

Solution

- In the given case patient is severely neutropenic and immunocompromised, so patient is prone for opportunistic infection.

- Based on the findings, i.e., catalase negative and oxidase negative with gram smear showed purple colour gram-positive organism that are in chains or pairs.

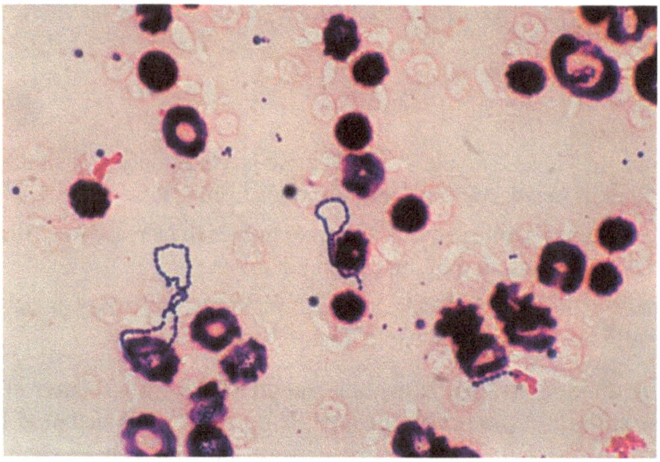

Gram smear of streptococcus

This image is a work of the Centers for Disease Control and Prevention, part of the United States Department of Health and Human Services, taken or made as part of an employee's official duties. As a work of the U.S. federal government, the image is in the public domain

- The image given in question is that of 'Ring precipitation test'. This test is positive for streptococcus.
- Streptococcus viridans is normally found in mouth and respiratory tract. It can cause bacteremia eating, toothbrushing, flossing and other minor trauma.
- Treatment for neutropenic patient getting bacteremia of Streptococcus viridans is 'Vancomycin'.
- For other infection it is penicillin.

13. 55 years old male underwent a prosthetic valve surgery 1 week ago. Later he tells doctor that he has to get his tooth extraction done cause his tooth cavity is really causing him pain. What do your doctor will advise this patient?

A. Dental procedures like tooth extraction are contraindicated after prosthetic valve surgery for 1 year

B. Ask his dentist to give Prophylactic antibody to prevent bacteremia and vegetative growth on prosthetic valve

C. Not to get tooth extraction at least for 6 months

D. No need for any preventive measure

Answer: B. Ask his dentist to give Prophylactic antibody to prevent bacteremia and vegetative growth on prosthetic valve

Solution

- Streptococcus viridans is normally found in mouth and respiratory tract so upon procedures like tooth extraction can cause transient bacteremia and eventually cause vegetative growth on prosthetic valve or damaged valve or congenitally diseased heart.
- They are generally non pathogenic but can cause endocarditis on already existing lesion.

14. 8 years old boy was brought to pediatrician by his parents with complain of generalised swelling specially on his feet and periorbital region and decreased urine for the last 2 days. Upon further taking history it was found that boy was having dark coloured urine along froth/foamy formation when he urinated. Parent of the patient told the doctor that for 1 week he is having sore throat along with impetigo (Image given below). Upon checking child's oxygen saturation it was found to be 90%. Doctor conducted few test that came to be positive. Identify the test conducted with the image given.

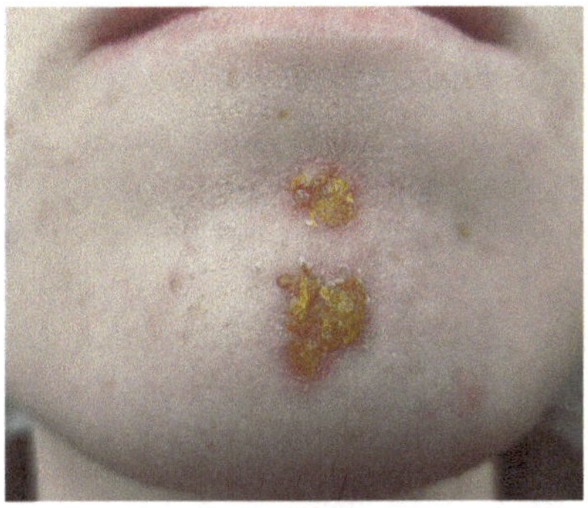

Impetigo

Source: Wikipedia; Author: James Heilman, MD; License: Creative Commons Attribution-ShareAlike 4.0 International license

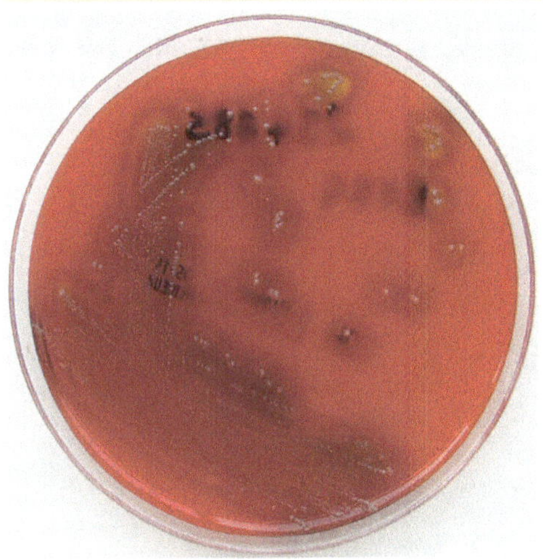

Test - 1

Source: Wikipedia; Author: Nathan Reading from Halesowen, UK
License: Creative Commons Attribution 2.0 Generic license

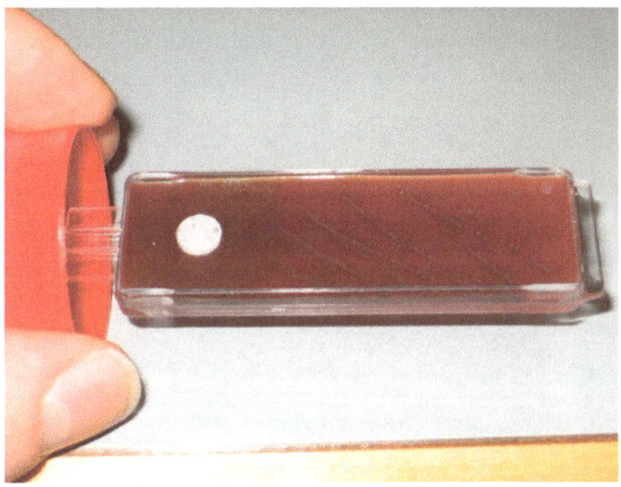

Test - 2

Source: Wikipedia; Author: Pöllö
License: Creative Commons Attribution 3.0 Unported license

A. Test-1: Pinpoint Beta hemolysis
   Test-2: Maxted observation Bacitracin sensitivity test

B. Test-1: Pinhead colonies beta hemolysis
   Test-2: CAMP test

C. Test-1: Alpha hemolysis
   Test-2: Pyrrolidonyl arylamidase (PYR)

D. Test-1: Gamma hemolysis

Test-2: Maxted observation Bacitracin sensitivity test

Answer: A. Test-1: Pinpoint beta hemolysis
Test-2: Maxted observation Bacitracin sensitivity test

Solution

- In this case symptoms like generalised edema, dark colored urine and foamy/froth after urinating with decrease in urine output is indicative towards Nephritic syndrome.
- Since the patient also had sore throat along with impetigo this is indicative towards Streptococcus infection. M type of streptococcus which causes glomerulonephritis is M1, M3, M49, M57. PSGN generally occurs 1-2 weeks after infection of untreated Streptococcus pyogenes.
- So the test that are shown in the image and which are specific for Streptococcus are: Test-1: beta hemolysis pin point colonies, Test-2: Maxted's observation sensitivity to Bacitracin.
- Another test which is specific for Streptococcus pyogenes is pyrrolidonyl-aryl-amidase activity (PYR) test positive.

15. 5 years old boy brought by his parents with complain of sore throat fever and malaise for 4 days. Also they give history of white coating on tongue which peeled off after few days leaving behind red swollen tongue (image given below).

Also there are red rashes and spots on body as given below. What is drug of choice for this patient?

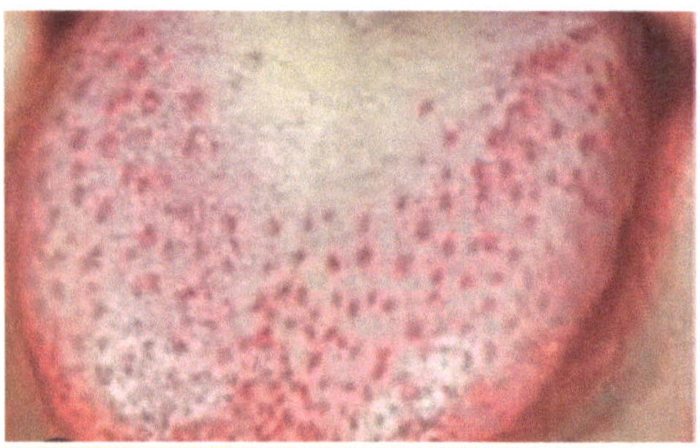

Source: Wikipedia; Author: Afag Azizova
License: Creative Commons Attribution-ShareAlike 3.0 Unported license

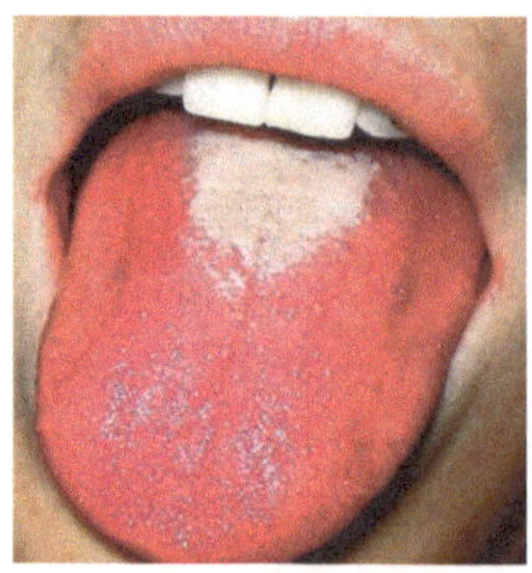

Source: Wikipedia; Author: Martin Kronawitter
License: Creative Commons Attribution-ShareAlike 2.5 Unported license

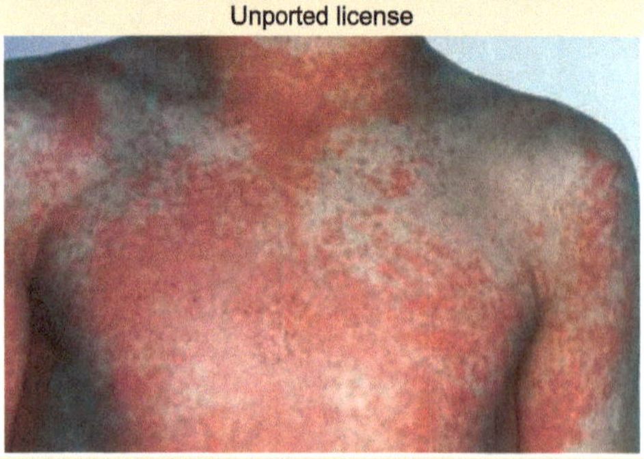

Source: Wikipedia; Author: The original uploader was Estreya at English Wikipedia
License: Creative Commons Attribution-ShareAlike 2.5 Unported license

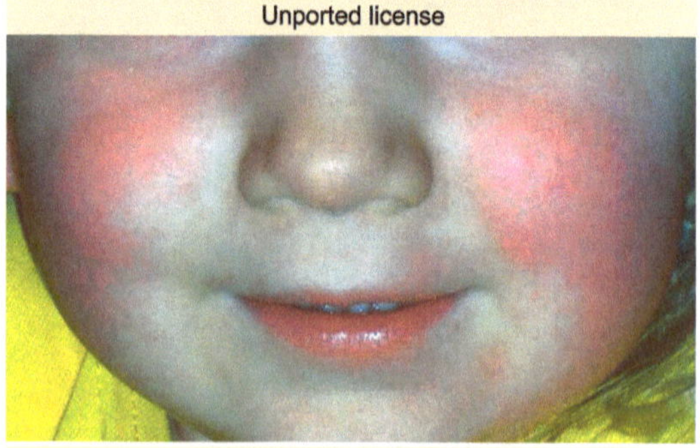

Source: Wikipedia, Author: Estreya at English Wikipedia | Permission=CC-BY-2.5; CC-BY-SA-2.5; License: Creative Commons Attribution-ShareAlike 4.0 Unported license

A. Oseltamivir

B. Ecanazole

C. Amphoteracin ointment

D. Beta lactam

Answer: D. Beta lactam

Solution

- The given case is that of Scarlet fever which is caused by Streptococcus pyogenes.
- Streptococcus is classified as 'Brown's classification' which is based upon hemolysis on blood agar pour plate culture as beta, alpha and gamma.
- Beta Hemolytic streptococcus is classified according to Lancefield serogrouping which is based upon 'c' carbohydrates in cell classification goes from A to V except I and J.
- Group A or streptococcus pyogenes is further classified as Griffith typing which is based upon M protein in cell wall.
- There are >120 M type of group A streptococcus.
- There are further sub typing on the basis of T and R protein.
- M protein is coded by 'emm' gene.

16. 8 years old boy was brought to pediatrician by his parents with complain of generalised swelling specially on his feet and periorbital region and decreased urine for last 2 days. Upon further taking history it was found that boy was having dark colored urine along froth/foamy formation when he urinated. Parent of the patient told the doctor that for 1 week he is having sore throat along with impetigo (image given below). Upon checking child's oxygen saturation it was found to be 90%. Doctor is suspecting Post Streptococcal Glomerulonephritis.What test should be performed to confirm diagnosis of PSGN?

A. ASO titre

B. Blood culture

C. Urine examination

Answer: A. ASO titre

Solution

- One of the toxins that are secreted by Streptococcus is 'Hemolysin' or 'Streptolysin'. These are of 2 types: SLO and SLS.

SLO

- It is oxygen labile, active in reduced state.
- Hemolysis only in pour plate culture.
- Produced by Group A,C,G streptococcus.
- It is leucocidal and cardiotoxic.
- In rheumatic fever and glomerulonephritis the diagnosis of streptococcus can be made by high levels of antibodies against Streptolysin O (SLO), i.e., anti Streptolysin O titration (ASO titre).

SLS

- Oxygen stable, active in both reduced and oxidised state.
- Hemolysis around surface colonies.

- For treatment of PSGN supportive treatment should be given with regular monitoring of kidney function, if infection still present then give antibiotics.

17. 70 years old patient comes with complain of progressive right knee swelling and pain for last 1 week. Patient informs that 1 month ago he tripped and landed on knee causing minor abrasion. Patient got total knee replacement surgery 5 years ago. The orthopedician conducts few tests on blood and synovial fluid specimen revealing it to be Streptococcus pyogenes. `Therefore doctor prescribed him Clindamycin and Penicillin G. But later that evening patient's condition deteriorated rapidly causing Tachycardia, sweating, hypotension eventually dying of Toxic Shock Syndrome. Which toxin is responsible for Toxic Shock Syndrome?

A. Scarlatiniform toxin/Dick/pyrogenic/erythrogenic
B. Enterotoxin
C. VMA
D. Hemolysin

Answer: A. Scarlatiniform toxin/Dick/pyrogenic/erythrogenic

18. Microbiologist was studying an organism with following characteristics gram-positive purple color cocci in chains or pair seen on gram smear. Forms beta Hemolytic pinpoint colonies on blood agar, catalase negative and oxidase negative. It shows positive ring precipitation test. What is the medical usage of this organism?

A. Streptokinase/Fibrinolysis produced by Group C and K streptococcus used for thrombolysis
B. Streptokinase/Fibrinolysis produced by Streptococcus pyogenes used for thrombolysis
C. Streptokinase/Fibrinolysis produced by Streptococcus viridans used for thrombolysis

Answer: A. Streptokinase/Fibrinolysis produced by Group C streptococcus (streptococcus equisimilus) and group K streptococcus

19. 26 years old primigravida female in her 35-week gestation comes for regular check up and doctor advises her to undergo rectal swabs and lower vaginal swab blood agar revealed beta Hemolytic pin point colonies. While on Islam's medium there is presence of orange pigment. What should be the following step in managing this patient?

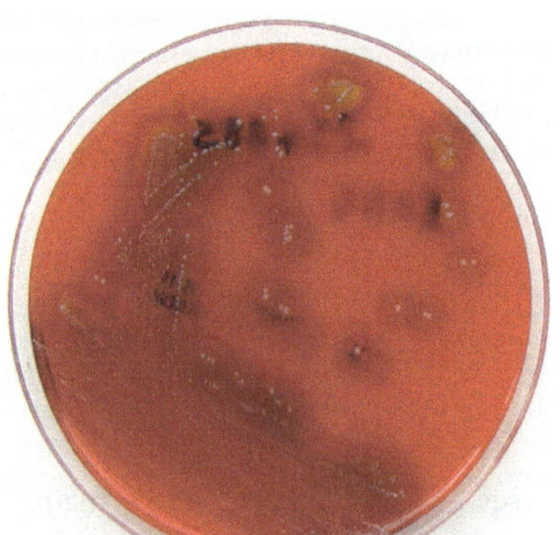

Pin point beta Hemolytic on Blood agar

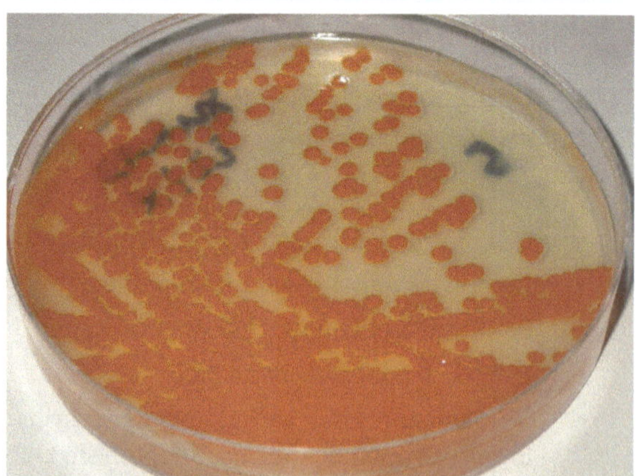

Orange pigment on Islam's or Granada medium

A. No need for any preventive measure or prophylaxis

B. Cesarean section at 36 weeks

C. Prophylactic antibiotic intrapartum penicillin

D. Streptomycin and kanamycin

Answer: C. Prophylactic antibiotic intrapartum penicillin

Solution

- In the given case patient undergoes routine check up to look for the presence of Streptococcus agalactiae which is part of normal flora of GIT and female genital urinary tract.
- If newborn gets infected with Streptococcus agalactiae then it may cause complication like Septicemia, Meningitis, pneumomia.
- To prevent this patient should be given prophylactic antibiotics like intrapartum penicillin.
- Option D Streptomycin and kanamycin should not be given as it can cause hearing loss.

20. 3 weeks old newborn was brought with complain of fever, focal seizure, signs of photophobia. Based on this doctor ask to get his blood and CSF culture done along with the following test shown below. Name the test shown below along with organism responsible for infant pathology.

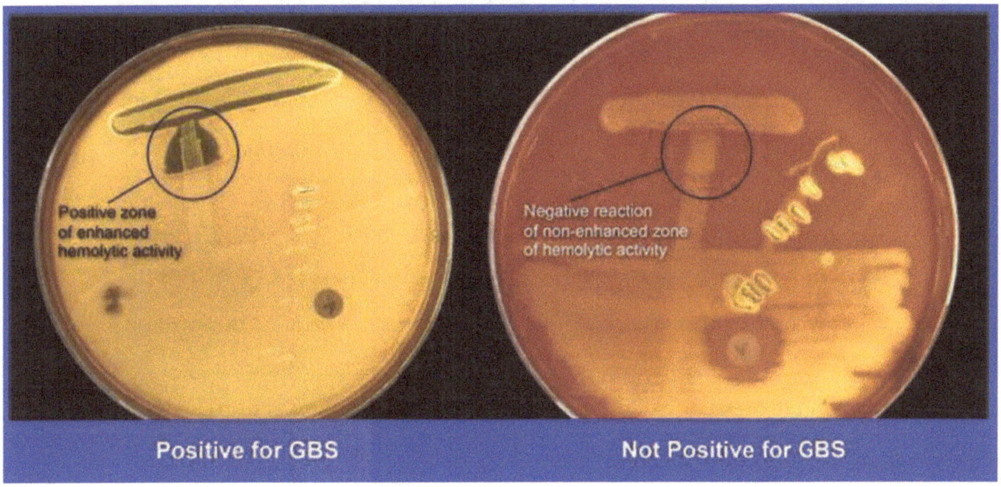

If the laboratory is not able to identify group-B streptococci (GBS) by the Lancefield grouping procedure, there are other microbiologic tests that can be used to identify GBS. This picture shows one of these tests. It is called the CAMP test. CAMP is an acronym for the authors of this test (Christie, Atkinson, Munch, Peterson). The CAMP test takes advantage of the capacity of GBS to produce this CAMP factor; most other hemolytic streptococci do not produce CAMP factor. This picture shows the growth and CAMP test of a GBS (Lt) and a group A Streptococcus (GAS) (Rt). On the top of the agar plate we have inoculated the plate with a Staphylococcus strain (horizontal streak). We then inoculated the GBS (on left) and GAS (on right) perpendicular to the "Staph" streak, making sure not to touch the two different organisms (Staph and Strep), but to come close to each other

A. Reverse CAMP test; Clostridium perfringens

B. Reverse CAMP test; Streptococcus agalactiae

C. CAMP test; Clostridium perfringens

D. CAMP test; Streptococcus agalactiae

Answer: D. CAMP test; Streptococcus agalactiae

Solution

- In this case infant is suffering from Meningitis infection which most probably got prenataly.
- The test that is depicted in image is that of CAMP test positive which is seen in case of Group B Streptococcus or Streptococcus agalactiae which is responsible for Meningitis in this patient.

21. 19 years old college going student suddenly starts having nausea, vomiting, watery diarrhea. He tells that he had milk and cereals for the breakfast. Upon conducting gram smear purple colored gram-positive cocci were seen which were catalase positive and oxidase negative, showed beta hemolysis and pin head colonies were seen on blood agar, tiny lactose fermenting colonies were seen on MacConkey medium and on nutrient agar it produced golden color pigment. Name this golden color pigment and incubation period for food poisoning caused by this organism.

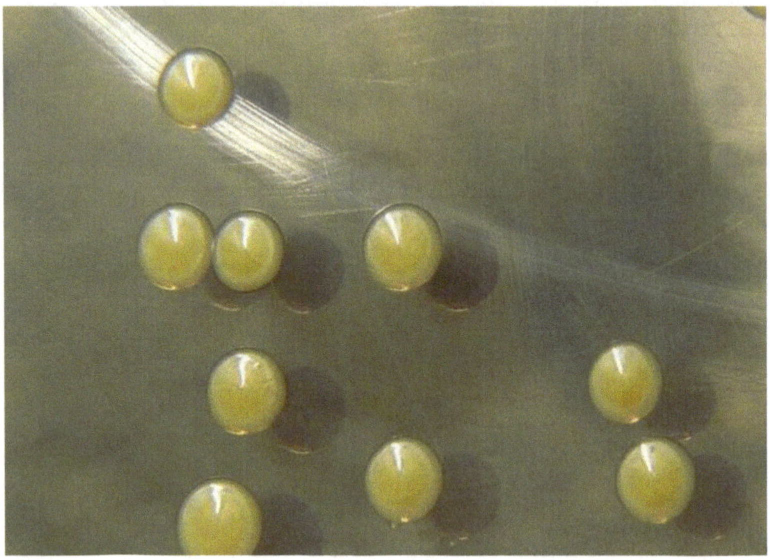

Source: Wikipedia; Author: Hans N; License: Creative Commons Attribution 3.0 Unported license

A. Hemolysin, 24 hours
B. Hemolysin, 12 hours
C. Staphyloxanthin, 6 hours
D. Coagulase, 6 hours

Answer: C. Staphyloxanthin, 6 hours

Solution

- The given case is that of Staphylococcus aureus food poisoning.
- Staphylococcus aureus gives pinhead colonies beta hemolysis on blood agar and on nutrient agar there is presence of gloden pigment, i.e., Staphyloxanthin. It is also said to have oil paint appearance.
- The toxin produced by Staphylococcus aureus that causes food poisoning is 'Enterotoxin'.
- Its heat stable resists 100°C for 30-40 minutes so can cause food poisoning even with cooked meal.
- In this case patient had milk and cereal for breakfast which could have been a source for this Staphylococcus aureus induced food poisoning.
- Incubation period for Staphylococcus aureus induced food poisoning is < 6 hours.

- Toxin produced by Staphylococcus aureus which is responsible for food poisoning is enterotoxin.
- Mechanism of action of enterotoxin is by stimulation of vagus and vomiting center.
- For treatment there is spontaneous resolution in 10-12 hours, no need of antibiotics.

22. Analyse the image below:

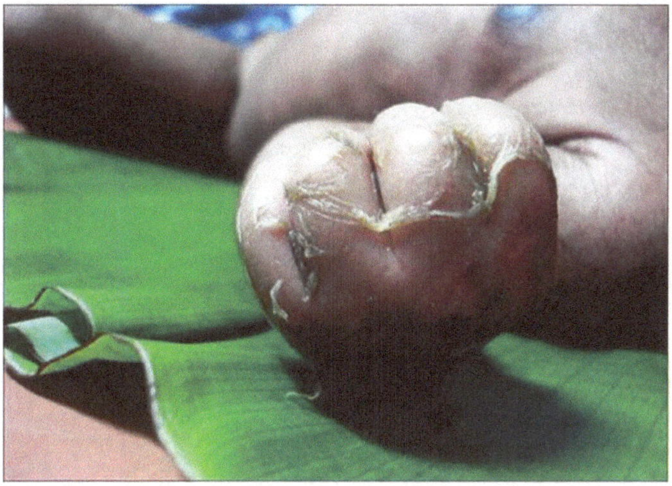

Which toxin is responsible for this condition and which layer of skin is affected?

A. Panton valentine leukocidin, Stratum corneum

B. Hemolysin, Stratum granulosum

C. Enterotoxin, Stratum corneum

D. Exfoliative/Epidermolytic toxin, Stratum granulosum

Answer: D. Exfoliative/Epidermolytic toxin, Stratum granulosum

Solution

- The given image is that of Ritter's disease or scalded skin syndrome. It is caused by Staphylococcus aureus which produces Exfoliative toxin or Epidermolytic toxin that proteolyse 'desmoglein-1' present in Stratum granulosum of neonates, young infants.
- **Diagnosis:** ELISA on serum for Exfoliative toxin.
- **Treatment**: Topical antibiotics.

23. 39 years old female is brought to Emergency room in state of confusion, with anxious look on face. Her husband said that she was feeling unwell for the last 10-12 hours. He denies of significant history. Upon examining her BP was 100/60, pulse 100 and was having tachycardia. Suspecting it to be a case of septic shock. Doctor ask to conduct blood, urine and stool culture. While inserting catheter for urine culture retained vaginal tampon was found. Upon conducting blood investigation pathogenic organism was Staphylococcus aureus. Which of the following blood agar colonies will we notice for Staphylococcus aureus?

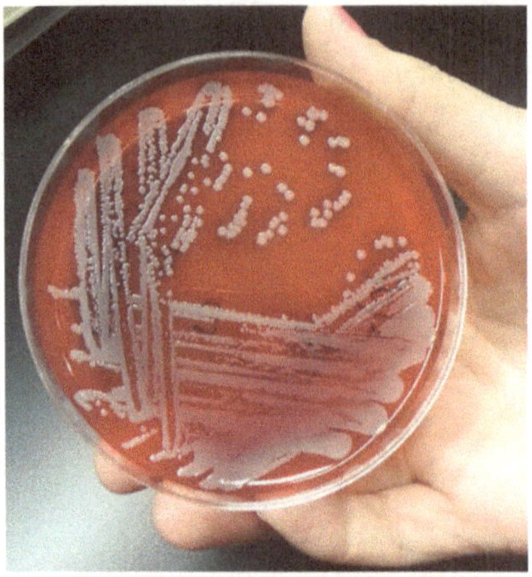

A.

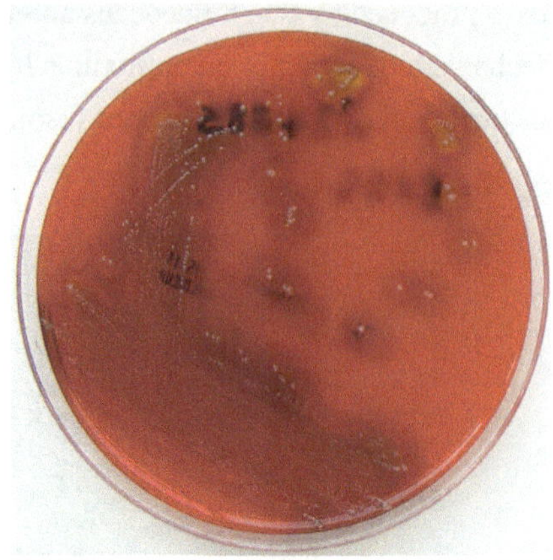

B.

C.

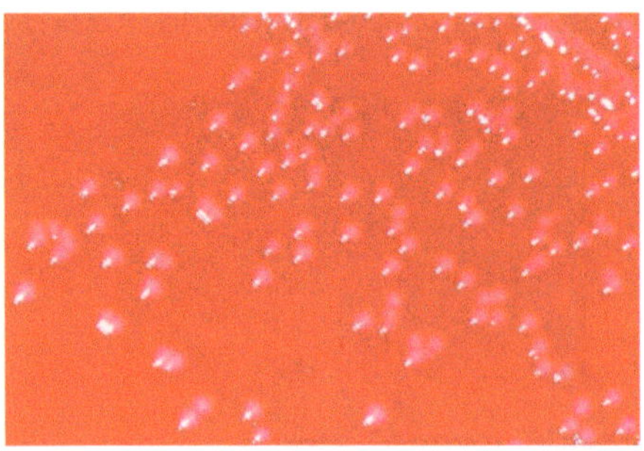

D.

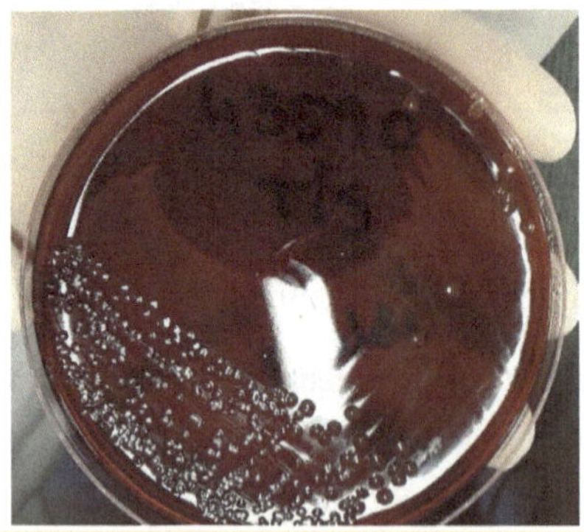

Answer: A.

24. 32 years old male presents to Emergency room with complain of gross hematuria. He has NOS associated history of increased frequency or urgency for urination along with burning sensation. There is no history of trauma or getting involved in activities like horse riding. Patient has a history of hypertension for last 6 years and have been on ACE inhibitor since then. Patient has a history of MRSA cutaneous infection for which incision and drainage was performed along with oral therapy with which patient was non compliant. On physical examination his vitals were: Pulse rate of 85, Blood Pressure of 192/101, fever was 100.2°C and respiratory rate of 18. There was no other remarkable findings. Based on this consulting doctor was highly suspecious for MRSA related glomerulonephritis and conducted serological test for MRSA, urine analysis and renal biopsy. The serological test came out to be positive, urine analysis showed the presence of proteinuria, dysmorphic RBC's also biopsy showed crescent formation in many of glomeruli. The consulting doctor decided to initiate therapy of giving Vancomycin to the patient. What is the biggest drawback of giving Vancomycin to such patient?

A. Vancomycin is not very effective against MRSA

B. Vancomycin is nephrotoxic and will cause further deterioration of patient's renal function

C. Vancomycin is hepatotoxic in nature

D. Vancomycin can cause encephalitis specially with high creatinine levels

Answer: B. Vancomycin is nephrotoxic and will cause further deterioration of patient's renal function

25. 3 years old child brought by her parents with the following presentation:

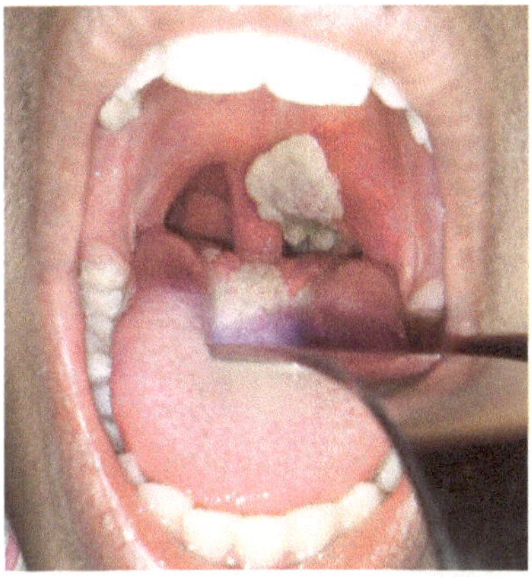

Source: Wikipedia; Author: User: Dileepunnikri
License: Creative Commons Attribution 3.0 Unported license

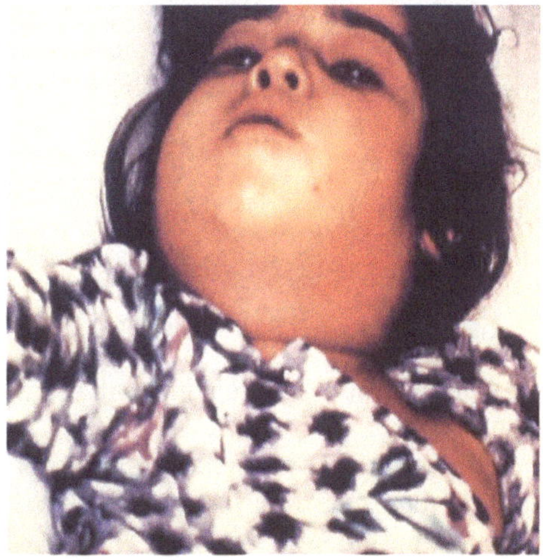

Suspecting it to be case of Corynebacterium diphtheria. What finding is expected on gram smear?

A. Purple colored gram-positive rod shaped Chinese letter appearance or cuneiform appearance

B. Gram-positive rod shaped bamboo stick appearance

C. Gram-negative rose pink spirals

D. Gram-negative pink color cocci in string or pair

Answer: A. Purple colored gram-positive rod shaped Chinese letter appearance or cuneiform appearance

Solution

- The given image is of Bull neck which is caused by corynebacterium diphtheria.
- Under gram smear Corynebacterium diphtheria is purple colored gram-positive rod shaped with Chinese letter arrangement or cuneiform appearance.

Biochemical Properties of Corynebacterium Diphtheria:

1. Catalase positive and oxidase negative.
2. Nitrate reduction test positive.
3. Urease test positive (helps to differentiate from C. ulcerans and C. pseudotuberculosis).
4. **Selective media**–Potassium tellurite media/hoyles agar/MacLeod downie tinsdale/cystine tellurite agar.

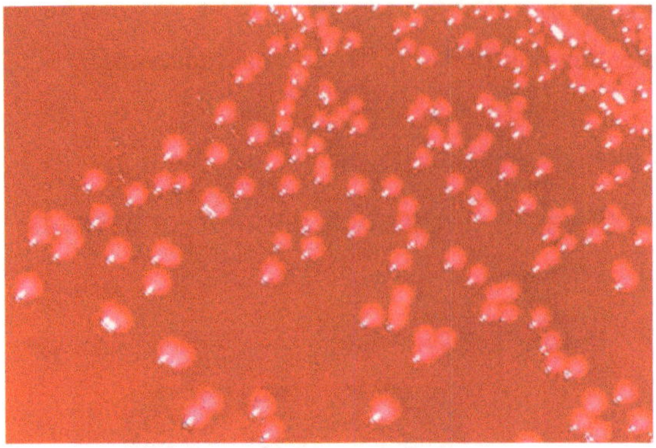

Hoyle medium-corynebacterium diphtheria growth

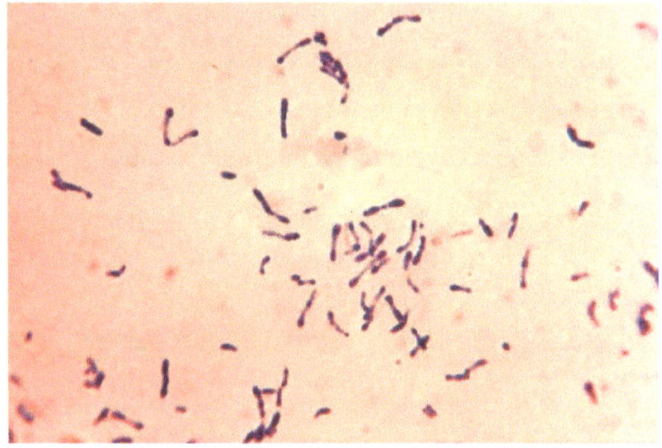

Gram smear

Diphtheria:

- **Reservoir**–Humans.
- **Peak age group**–2-5 years.
- **Incubation period**–3-4 days.
- **Complication**–Most common myocarditis around 7-10 days which manifest as AV block.

26. 56 years old male presents with complain of fever and malaise. He underwent orthopedic transplant surgery 3 days ago. Which of the following is correct for the most likely organism to cause this pathology?

A. Non-hemolytic

B. Novobiocin resistant

C. Drug of choice against this organism is penicillin

D. Generally found in GIT and female urinary tract

Answer: A. Non-hemolytic

Solution

- Most common cause for bacteremia/infection after orthopedic transplant surgery is Staphylococcus epidermis.
- Most common cause for lumbar puncture associated meningitis.
- Most common cause for dialysis associated peritonitis.
- It is associated with post intervention infection such as IV cannula, CSF shunt, prosthetic valve surgery and catheter.
- It is associated with endocarditis, wound infection, sinus infection, boils.

- Its gram-positive facultative anaerobe.
- It is part of normal flora of skin.
- It is part of CONS (Coagulase Negative Staphylococcus).
- It is multi drug resistant.
- Drug of choice is clindamycin + penicillinase resistant penicillin.
- It is Novobiocin sensitive.

27. 18 years old young female presents with complain of burning micturition, urgency, frequency in urination for the last 3 days. Doctor prescribes patient to undergo urine culture, it was found that she was having purple color gram-positive cocci which was catalase positive and oxidase negative, Coagulase negative, Novobiocin resistant. Name the organism responsible for patient condition.

A. E. coli
B. Proteus
C. Streptococcus agalactiae
D. Staphylococcus aureus
E. Staphylococcus saprophyticus

Answer: E. Staphylococcus saprophyticus

Solution

Option A. E. coli: It is gram-negative pink color rod shaped on gram smear. So it is excluded. It is catalase positive and oxidase negative since it is part of Enterobacteriaceae.

Option B. Proteus comes under classification of Enterobacteriaceae and is catalase positive and oxidase negative, urease test is positive, nitrate reduction test is also positive. Hydrogen disulfide gas production on sugar fermentation, swarming on blood agar, PPA test positive.

Option C. Streptococcus agalactiae is beta hemolytic, CAMP test positive, Catalase negative and oxidase negative, produces orange color pigment on Islam's or Granada medium.

Option D. Staphylococcus aureus is gram-positive cocci catalase positive and oxidase negative which is both slide and tube Coagulase positive, produces golden colour Staphyloxanthin pigment on nutrient agar, Lysostaphin sensitive.

Option E. Staphylococcus saprophyticus: It is a part of Coagulase negative staphylococcus. Catalase positive and oxidase negative.

- It is generally associated with Urinary Tract Infection in young females.
- It is also known to cause honeymoon cystitis.
- Novobiocin resistant.
- UTI caused by staphylococcus saprophyticus is generally diagnosed 1-2 weeks after marriage.

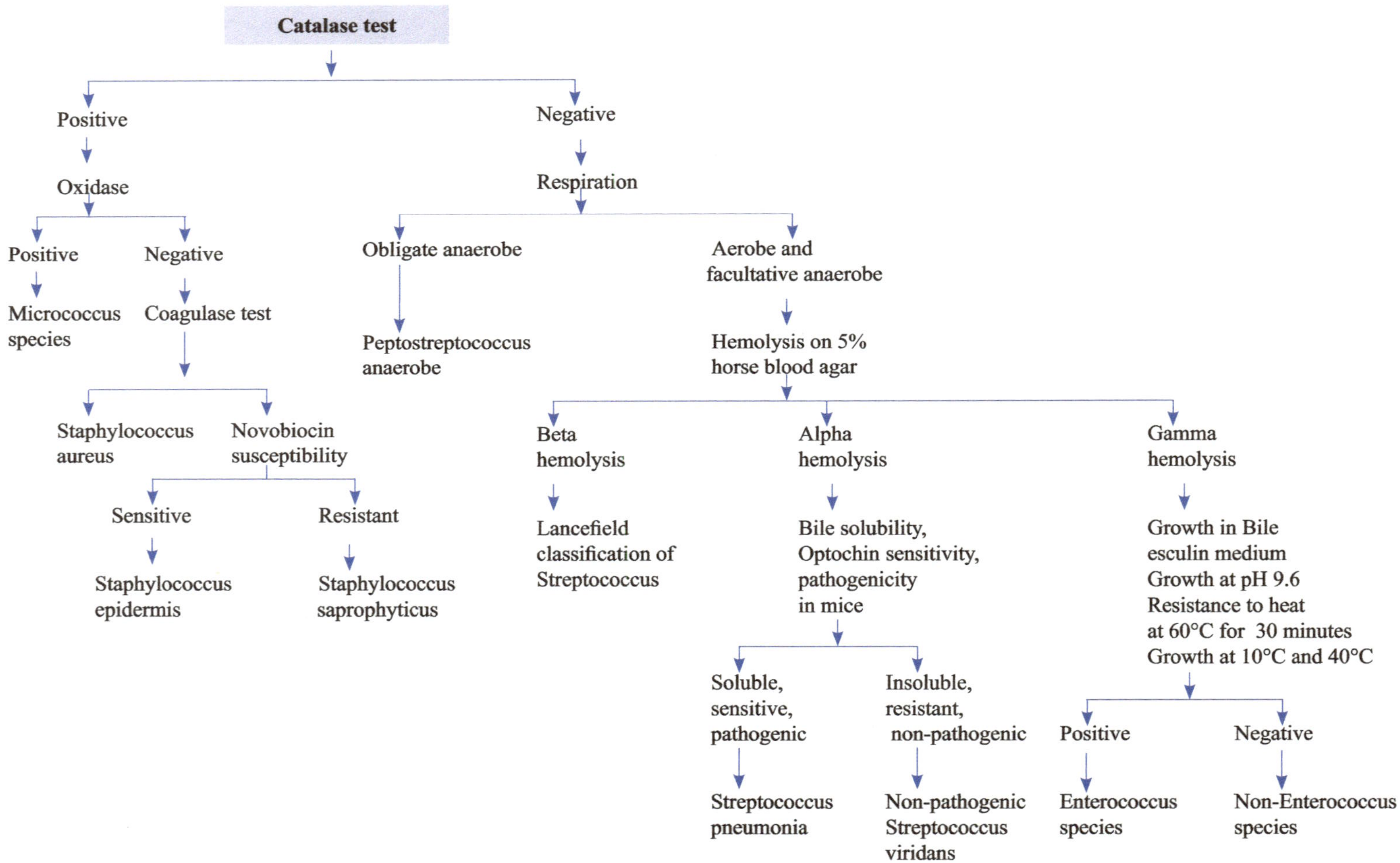

Note:

B Beta hemolytic–Complete hemolysis.

A Alpha hemolytic–Partial hemolysis.

G Gamma hemolytic–Incomplete hemolysis.

28. 68 years old male comes with complain of fever, cough for the last 4 days and difficulty in breathing and shortness of breath for the last 2 days. His breathing is rapid and shallow. He has hypertension for the last 38 years and Diabetes mellitus-2 for the last 35 years. He is currently on captopril and thiazide diuretic for hypertension. Along with that he takes insulin 3 times a day for DM-2. Doctor sends patient sputum for culture and other test whose images are shown below. Correctly identify the names of these 2 tests:

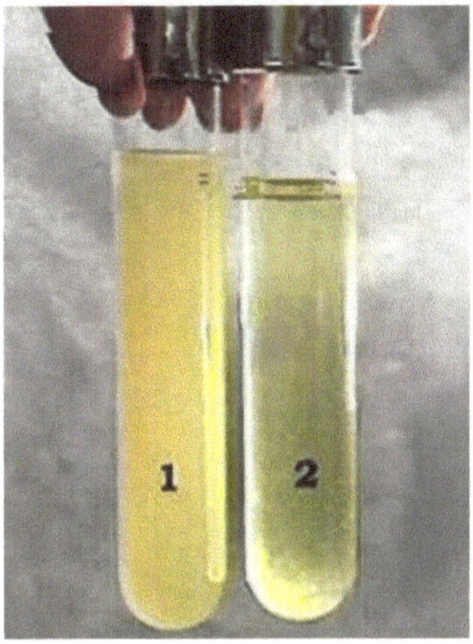

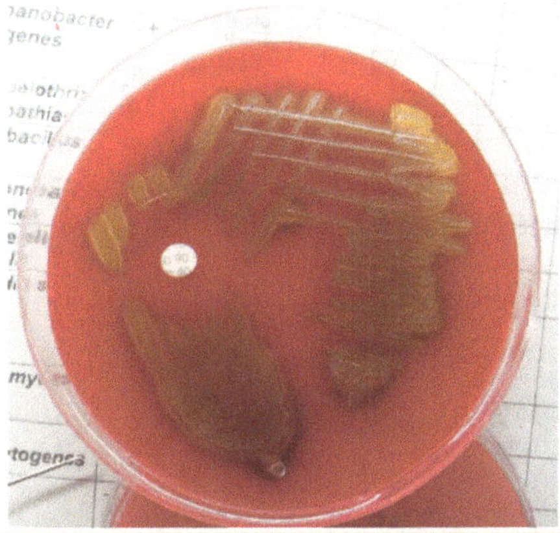

Source: Wikipedia; Author: User: GS Bhalla License: Creative Commons Attribution 4.0 International license

A. Bile solubility test; Blood agar alpha hemolysis with optochin sensitivity

B. Bile solubility test; Blood agar beta hemolysis with optochin sensitivity

C. Tube coagulase test; Blood agar beta hemolysis with novobiocin sensitivity

D. Tube coagulase test; Blood agar beta hemolysis with bacitracin sensitivity

Answer: A. Bile solubility test; Blood agar alpha hemolysis with optochin sensitivity

Solution

- The given image is of bile solubility, Streptococcus pneumoniae is lysed by bile. The other image is that Alpha hemolysis with optochin sensitivity seen in case of Streptococcus pneumoniae.

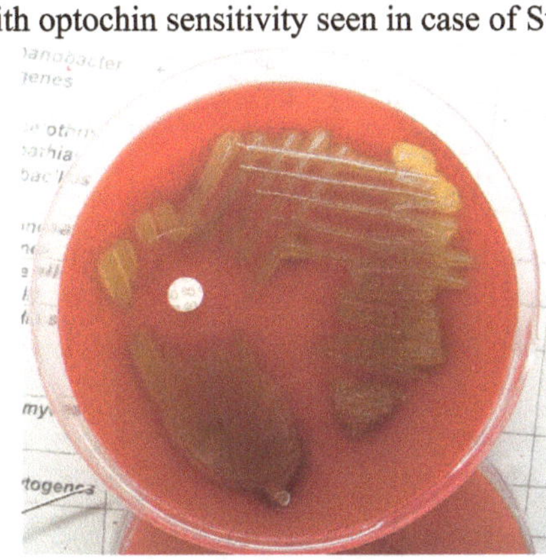

Streptococcus pneumoniae culture on blood agar showing optochin sensitivity

Source: Wikipedia; Author: User: GS Bhalla; License: Creative Commons Attribution 4.0 International license

- Streptococcus pneumoniae gives 'Draughtsman appearance' or 'Carrom Coin Colonies' on Blood agar. After 24-48 hours there are young Alpha hemolytic colonies with flattened-depressed centers.
- Streptococcus pneumoniae is most common causative organism for lobar pneumonia.

29. 28 years old male was brought to Emergency room with complain of altered mental status along with confusion for the last 12 hours. He was also having headache, fever, vomit, cough, shortness of breath and difficulty in breathing for the last 2 days. He has a medical history of HIV along with uncontrolled Diabetes mellitus-2. Doctor conducts gram smear with blood culture and Lumbar puncture for CSF study revealing purple colored Gram-positive cocci in pairs, lanceolate (flame shaped), Blood culture showed alpha hemolysis Carrom Coin Appearance Lumbar puncture had increased opening pressure, elevated proteins, decrease glucose, increase neutrophils. Based on this doctor made diagnosis of Streptococcus pneumoniae and started penicillin which soon proved to be ineffective what should be next drug of choice?

A. Macrolides
B. Cephalosporins
C. Fluoroquinolones

Answer: A. Macrolides

Solution

- Given description is that of Streptococcus pneumoniae which is known to cause pathologies like pneumonia meningitis, otitis media.
- It is gram-positive cocci which on gram smear appears as purple coloured cocci appearing in pairs, lanceolated, flame shaped.

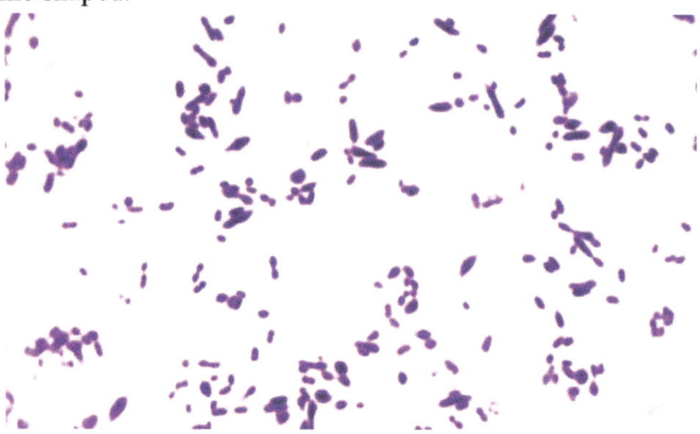

Streptococcus pneumoniae gram smear

- Its capsule is polysaccharide in nature and is considered one of the main virulence factor which prevents phagocytosis.
- On blood agar it cause alpha hemolysis (partial hemolysis) which has draughtsman/carrom coin appearance.

Biochemical Reactions:

B Bile solubility.

I Inulin fermenter.

O Optochin sensitive.

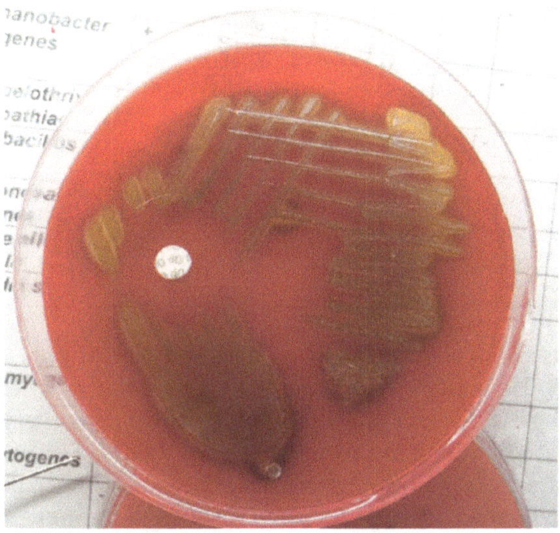

Source: Wikipedia; Author: User: GS Bhalla; License: Creative Commons Attribution 4.0 international license

Quellung Reaction or Neufeld Test:

- On the basis of capsule there are more than 90 serotypes of Streptococcus pneumoniae.
- Quellung is the German word for "swelling" and describes the microscopic appearance of pneumococcal or other bacterial capsules after their polysaccharide antigen has combined with a specific antibody. The antibody usually comes from serum taken from an immunized laboratory animal. As a result of this combination and precipitation of the large, complex molecule formed, the capsule appears to swell, because of increased surface tension and its outlines become clearly demarcated.
- It is used to identify the serotype of Streptococcus pneumoniae.

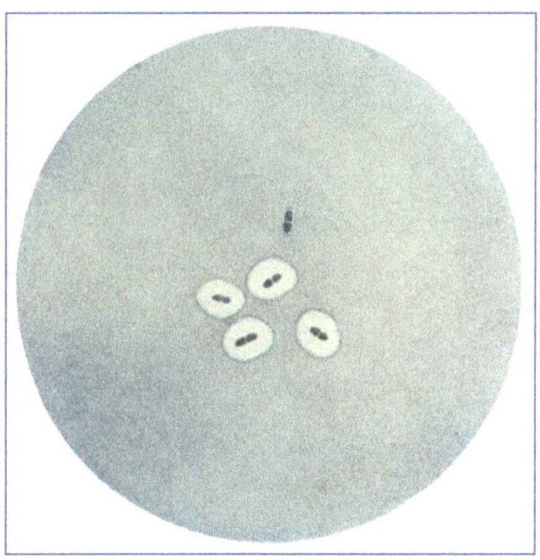

Quellung reaction or Neufeld test

- The antibody produced are serotype specific which is based upon polysaccharidal capsule.
- Certain serotypes of pneumococcus are resistant to penicillin due to modification of Penicillin Binding Protein to Penicillin Binding Protein 2b.
- So, drug of choice for penicillin resistant pneumococci is 'Macrolide'.

Type of bacteria	*Antibiotics that are resistant*
Anaerobic bacteria	Aminoglycosides
Aerobic bacteria	Metronidazole
Gram-negative bacteria	Vancomycin
Klebsiella	Ampicillin
Pseudomonas	Sulphonamide, Tetracycline, Chloramphenicol, Trimethoprim
Enterococci	Aminoglycosides and all cephalosporins
Mycoplasma	Cephalosporins

30. 48 years old presents with complain of fever, neck stiffness altered sensorium and photophobia for the last 10 hours. He underwent splenectomy 18 years ago when he met with Road Traffic Accident traumatising his spleen. Patient is smoking one packet every day for last 28 years. He is suffering from uncontrolled Diabetes despite of taking 3 dose of insulin every day. He has a recent history of returning from Hajj pilgrimage. Upon examination petechial/purpuric rash were found on lower limb, his limbs were cold, Heart rate 110 beats per minute, Blood Pressure 110/70.

Considering patient's condition doctor orders for lumbar puncture for CSF study and blood culture. Which of the following is correct regarding organism causing patient's pathology?

A. Gram-positive, diplococci

B. Catalase positive and oxidase negative

C. No prophylaxis is recommended for household contacts, Health care workers exposed to respiratory secretions

D. Reservoir–Humans, carriage site–Nasopharynx, Transmission–Airborne droplet of nasopharyngeal secretion

Answer: D. Reservoir–Humans, carriage site–Nasopharynx, Transmission–Airborne droplet of nasopharyngeal secretion

Solution

- The given case is that of Neisseria meningitis which is 'Gram-negative' diplococci which is 'Lens shaped or half moon shaped'.

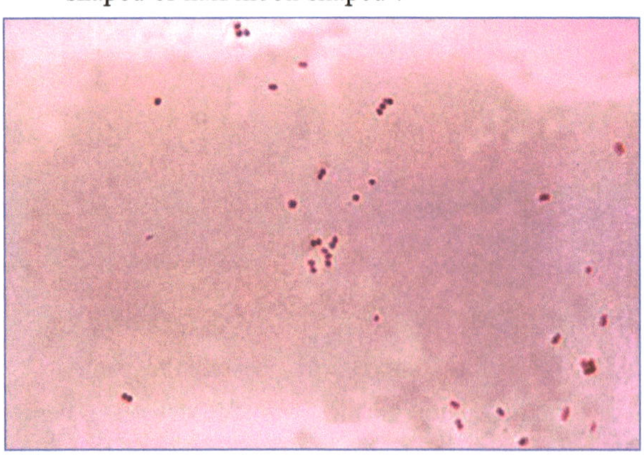

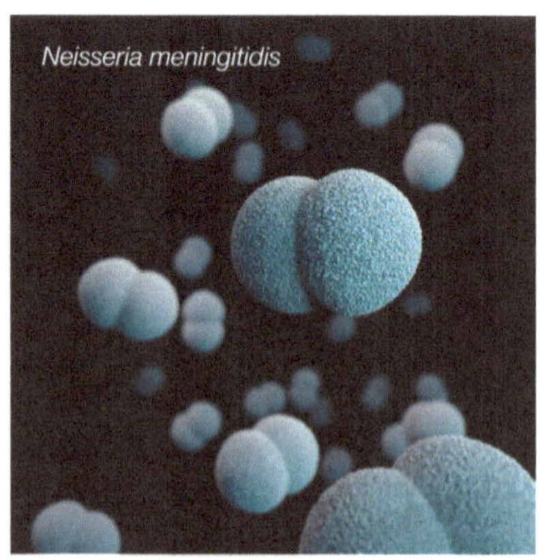

Gram smear pink color gram-negative 'Lens shaped or half moon shaped'

Biochemical Reactions:

- Catalase positive.
- Oxidase positive.
- Utilises sugar–all species utilise glucose except for Neisseria sicca which utilise sucrose and Neisseria lactamica which utilise lactose.
- Selective media for Neisseria 'Thayer-Martin'.
- Thayer-Martin medium is chocolate agar which have been modified to be selective for Neisseria meningitidis and Neisseria gonorrhoeae bus adding following antibiotics:
  1. **Vancomycin**–Inhibit most gram-positive bacteria.
  2. **Colistin**–Inhibit most gram-negative bacteria except Neisseria.
  3. **Nystatin or anisomycin**–Inhibit yeast growth.

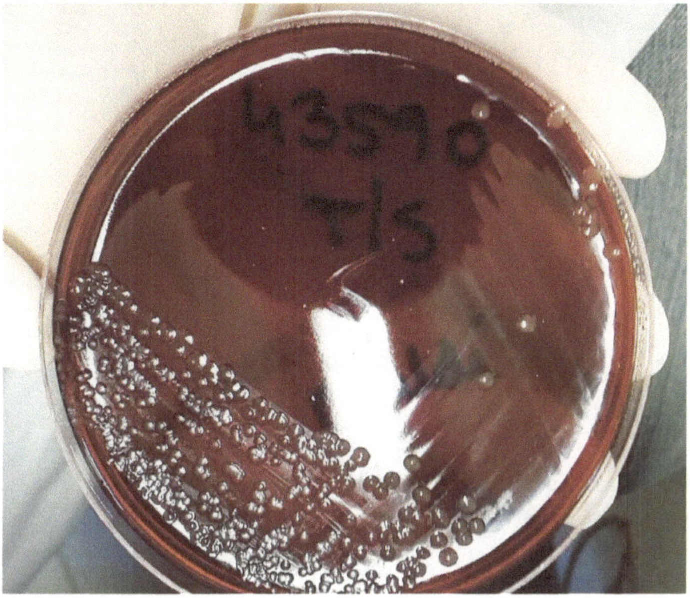

Thayer-Martin medium for Neisseria growth

Source: Wikipedia; Author: Xishan 01; License:Creative Commons Attribution 3.0 Unported license

- Chocolate agar contains Red Blood Cell that have been lysed by slowly heating to 80°C.
- Modified Thayer-Martin media or New York City media is same as Thayer-Martin media with addition of trimethoprim.
- Advantage of adding Trimethoprim is it inhibit swarming growth pattern of 'Proteus' making it more selective.

Epidemiology of Meningococcal:

- Reported all over the world with maximum cases coming from Mediterranean belt and Sub-Saharan Africa.
- **Transmission**–Airborne droplet of nasopharyngeal secretion.
- **Reservoir**–Human; Carriage site–Nasopharynx.
- Generally seen in places of overcrowding like dormitory, Hajj pilgrimage, refugees camp.

Risk Factors for Neisseria Associated Meningococcal Disease:

1. Smokers.
2. Recent viral infection.
3. Splenectomized.
4. Travellers to meningitis belt.
5. Infection with mycoplasma pneumoniae.
6. Hypogammaglobulinemia.
7. Terminal complement factors deficiency (C6-C9).

- Generally it is known to cause Meningitis or meningococcemia.
- **Symptoms**–Fever, headache, neck rigidity, photophobia, petechial or purpuric rash.

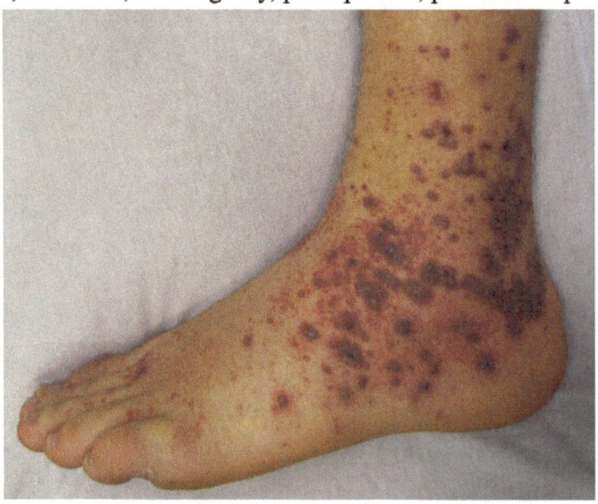

Petechial or purpuric rash seen in patient suffering from Neisseria meningitidis

Source: Wikipedia; Author: James Heilman, MD; License: Creative Commons Attribution 3.0 Unported license

Complications:

- Most common–Scaring of necrotic skin lesion.
- Neurological complication like deafness and psychological complication.

Treatment:

- First choice third generation Cephalosporins (IV) ceftriaxone or cefotaxime for one week. Blood or CSF becomes negative within 24 hours.
- If patient allergic to cephalosporins then give Chloramphenicol.

Prophylaxis is recommended for:

- Household contacts of patients.
- Health care workers directly exposed to respiratory secretions.
- **For adults**–Ciprofloxacin, Ceftriaxone, Rifampicin.
- **For pregnant women**–Only give Ceftriaxone.
- **For children**–Rifampicin or Ceftriaxone.

Note:

Post splenectomy patients are at risk of being infected by encapsulated organisms because capsule serves as anti-phagocytic virulence factor so to clear these organisms from body they underwent opsonisation and then cleared of by spleen but in asplenic patients that is not possible, therefore prone for getting infected by encapsulated organisms.

Examples: Pseudomonas aeruginosa, Streptococcus pneumoniae, Haemophilus influenzae type B, Neisseria meningitidis, E. coli, Salmonella, Klebsiella pneumoniae and group B Streptococcus, Bacillus anthracic, yersinia pestis, Cryptococcus neoformans.

31. 34 years old is brought to Emergency room with complain of pain in upper limb and lower limb along with nausea, vomiting and generalised weakness for 1 day. He was brought in confused state. Upon taking history it was found that his wife was suffering from Neisseria meningitidis infection for the last 1 week, being a household contact patient was advised to take prophylaxis for Neisseria meningitidis with which he was not compliant. He has a history of undergoing splenectomy after getting in Road Traffic Accident 16 years ago. His vitals were unstable pulse 95 beats per minute, blood pressure 110/55. On examination presence of petechial rash were seen on upper and lower limb. His limbs were cold and pale. Name the condition patient is suffering from.

A. Waterhouse-Friderichsen Syndrome (WFS)

B. Water can perineum

C. EHEC related Hemolytic Uremic Syndrome

Answer: A. Waterhouse-Friderichsen syndrome (WFS)

Solution

- In the given case person is suffering from Waterhouse-Friderichsen Syndrome.
- As given in the question patient's wife suffering from Neisseria meningitidis making her husband prone for getting infected specially since he is asplenic.
- When patient infected with Neisseria meningitidis he can have severe endotoxemia that will cause increase vascular permeability along with activation of coagulation pathway causing poor peripheral perfusion and causing symptoms like cold limbs, tachycardia, tachypnea.
- When it is severe disseminated intravascular coagulation along with endotoxic shock with multiple organ failure can occur. This is called Waterhouse-Friderichsen syndrome.
- Patient infected with Neisseria meningitidis can have post Meningococcal reactive disease due to deposition of immune complex and symptoms will be:
  - o Fever + arthritis (most common); or
  - o Fever + maculopapular rash/vasculitis rash; or
  - o Fever + iritis.

32. One week old male newborn starts having purulent conjunctival purulent discharge along with high grade of chemosis as shown in the image. Child was born by normal vaginal delivery. Doctor sends the purulent discharge and conjunctival scraping for giemsa staining and culture revealing presence pink color gram-negative bean/kidney shaped diplococci along with round convex or umbonate colonies. Which of following is correct for the organism?

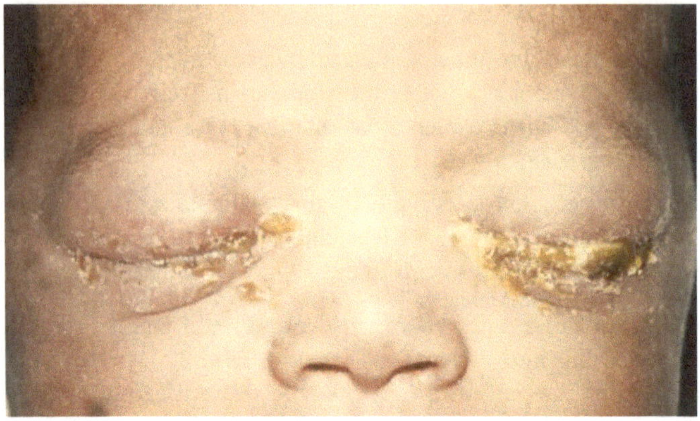

Content Provider(s): CDC/J. Pledger; License: Creative Commons Attribution 3.0 Unported license

A. Capsulated organism
B. Cause Waterhouse-Friderichsen syndrome
C. Cause watercan perineum
D. Catalase positive and oxidase negative

Answer: C. Cause watercan perineum

Solution

- Newborn is suffering from ocular gonorrhoeae. Which he most likely would have got from infected maternal tract during delivery.
- Gram smear–pink color gram-negative kidney or bean.
- Blood agar culture shows round, convex, umbonate colonies.

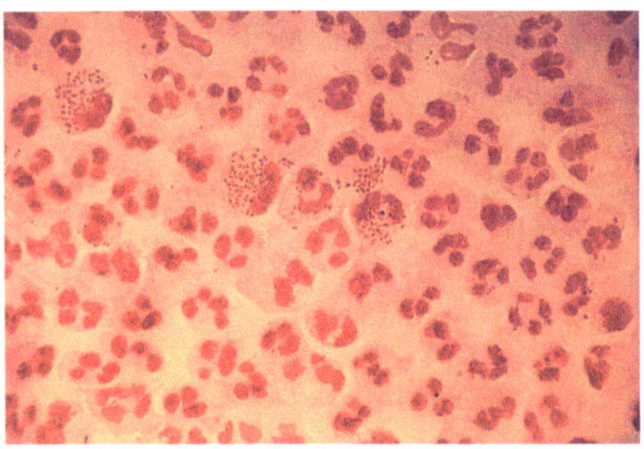

Gram smear of Neisseria gonorrhoeae

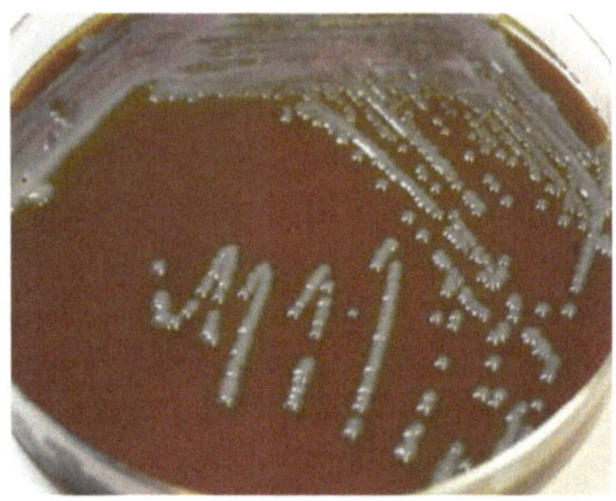

Round convex or umbonate colonies on blood agar

Biochemical Properties:

- Catalase positive and Oxidase positive utilise only glucose.
- It is non capsulated organism unlike meningococcus which is capsulated organism.

33. 35 years old female visits gastroenterologist with a complain of pain right upper quadrant for the last 2 weeks which has progressively increased. She denied use of OCP's for the last 6 months. She has a history of mucopurulent discharge and pain during coital activity. She has a history of multiple sex partners. Suspecting it to be a case of Pelvic Inflammatory Disease, doctor sends specimen for staining and culture. Results image are given below. Name the pathological organism and its drug of choice.

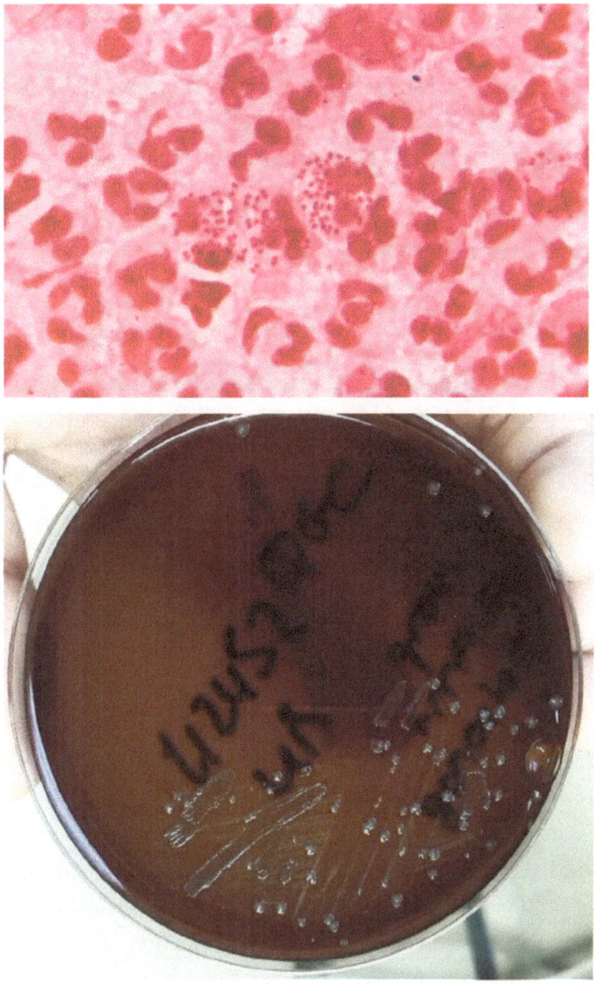

Modified New York agar medium showing round, convex or umbonate colonies

A. Chlamydia trachomatis, Azithromycin

B. Neisseria gonorrhoeae, Ceftriaxone

C. Gardnerella vaginalis, Metronidazole

D. E. coli, Penicillin

Answer: B. Neisseria gonorrhoeae, Ceftriaxone

Solution

- This is the case of Pelvic Inflammatory Disease which is caused by Neisseria gonorrhoeae advancing into Fitz-Hugh-Curtis syndrome.
- Fitz-Hugh-Curtis syndrome is caused by PID due to Neisseria gonorrhoeae or Chlamydia trachomatis.
- In Fitz-Hugh-Curtis syndrome there is inflammation of liver capsule along with adhesion formation resulting in right upper quadrant pain.

- Chlamydia trachomatis is obligate intracellular organism so Gram staining can't help us to visualise Chlamydia trachomatis.
- The given image of Gram stain shows pink color from negative diplococci that is kidney or bean shaped.
- Its cultured on modified New York City agar forming round, convex or umbonate colonies.

Biochemical Properties:

- Catalase positive and oxidase positive.
- It utilises glucose.
- **Treatment:** Drug of choice third generation Cephalosporins–Ceftriaxone.

34. 44 years old presents with complain of arthritis maculopapular rash, Tenosynovitis for the last 1 week. Based on patient history and examination doctor was suspicious of Neisseria infection but was not sure whether it is Neisseria gonorrhoeae or Neisseria meningitidis. Which of the following tests are most helpful for differentiating between Neisseria gonorrhoeae and Neisseria meningitidis?

A. Culture on Wilson and Blair Bismuth sulphite agar

B. CAMP test

C. Catalase and oxidase test

D. Maltose fermentation

Answer: D. Maltose fermentation

Solution

- Neisseria meningitidis can cause the complication like arthritis, maculopapular rash and Tenosynovitis as part of post Meningococcal Reactive disease due to deposition of immue complexes.
- While Neisseria gonorrhoeae can develop same complications as a part of Disseminated gonococcal infection.
- Best test to differentiate between gonorrhoeae and meningitidis is Maltose fermentation.
- N. meningitidis utilises glucose and Maltose.
- N. gonorrhea utilise glucose.

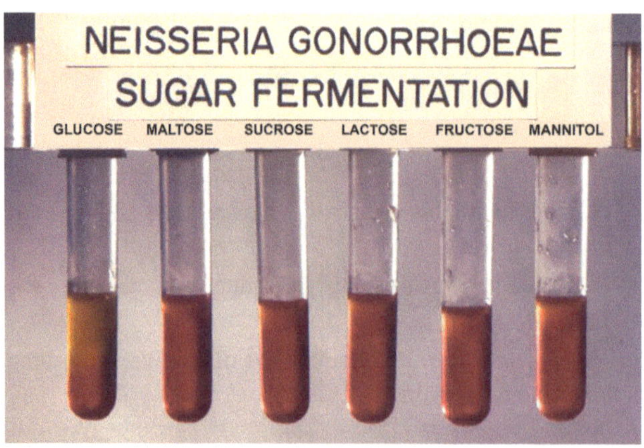

35. 13 years old male is brought to Emergency room in state of confusion along with complain of neck stiffness, photophobia for the last 6 hours. Diagnosis of Neisseria meningitidis was made after performing Polymerase chain reaction (PCR) and latex agglutination.Vaccine given to the patient to prevent Neisseria meningitidis contains which of the following components?

A. Outer membrane proteins for all serotypes

B. Capsular antigen for all serotypes

C. Capsular antigen for serotypes A, C, W and Y while for serotype B it is outer membrane protein as antigen

D. Outer membrane proteins for serotypes A, C, W and Y and capsular antigen for serotype B

Answer: C. Capsular antigen for serotypes A, C, W and Y while for serotype B it is outer membrane protein as antigen

Solution

- Neisseria meningitidis is divided into 13 serotypes on the basis of capsular antigen.
- Out of 13 serotypes, 6 of them causes human disease, i.e., serotypes A, B, C, X, Y, W.
- As far as vaccine is concerned capsular antigen are used for serotypes A,C,W,Y except serotype B Neisseria meningitidis.
- Capsular antigen is not used for type B serotype of Neisseria meningitidis because it shows molecular mimicry with fetal neural cell therefore for serotype B Neisseria meningitidis vaccine we use outer membrane protein as antigen.

36. 66 years old female was brought to Emergency room in state of confusion with severe abdominal distension followed by severe pain 2 hours ago. In accordance to Numeric Pain Scale it was 9/10. Doctor ask for bed side X-ray which revealed following findings.

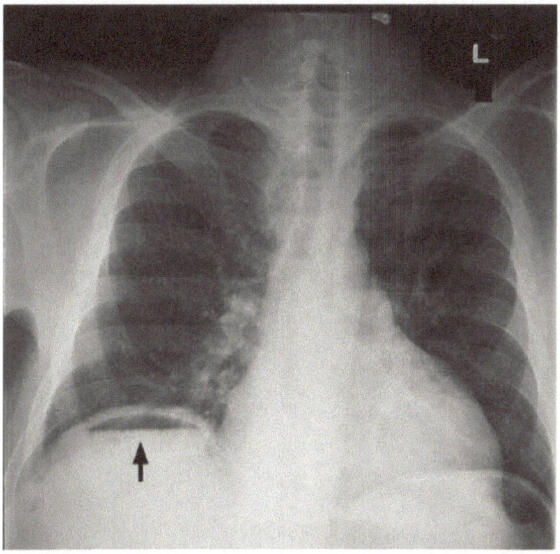

Source: http://clinical cases.blogspot.com/2004/03/bloody-ascites-and-gas-under-diaphragm.html, Wikipedia

Relatives of patient tells that she was having watery diarrhea along with fever and malaise for the last 1 week. She has a history of visiting to dentist for her Root Canal Treatment for which she was given multiple antibiotics. After initial treatment patient was clinically stable doctor decided to conduct colonoscopy ending up getting the following findings.

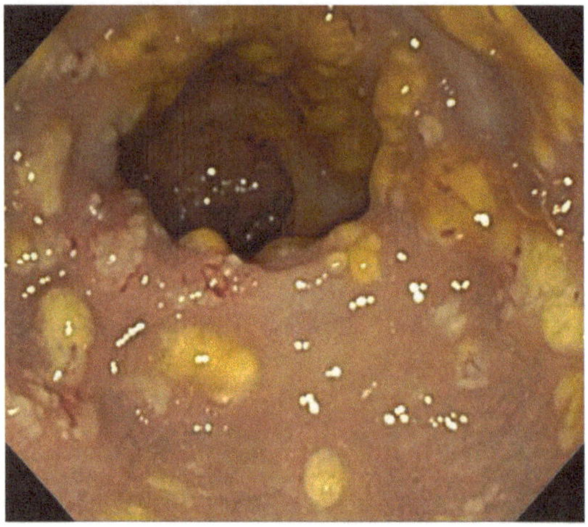

Colonoscopy findings of patient

Source: Wikipedia; Author: Samir; License: Creative Commons Attribution 3.0 Unported license

Which of the following is correct regarding patient's condition?

A. Organism responsible for patient's condition produces Botulinum toxin
B. Organism responsible for patient's condition has rod shaped appearance
C. Organism responsible for patient's condition is not part of GIT normal flora
D. Organism responsible for patient's condition produces sub terminal spores

Answer: B. Organism responsible for patient's condition has rod shaped appearance

Solution

- Based on patient's condition it is most likely that she is suffering from antibiotic associated clostridium difficile infection causing watery diarrhea eventually leading on to causing complication like megacolon and eventually perforation.
- Clostridium difficile is gram-positive, spore forming organism which has rod shaped appearance.

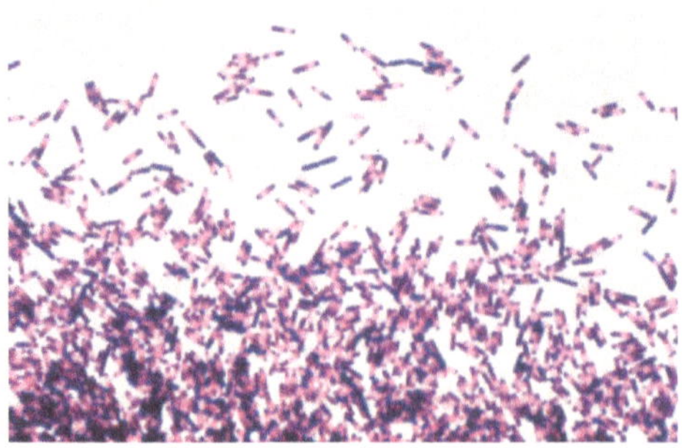

Gram smear showing gram-positive rod shaped Clostridium difficile

- Clostridium difficile is found in GI flora of certain individuals but do not cause disease as it is kept in check by other organism of GI flora.
- But sometimes due to excessive use of antibiotics as in this patient had taken antibiotics for Root Canal Treatment by her dentist which results in loss of normal GI flora and causing unchecked excessive growth of Clostridium difficile.
- Clostridium difficile produces Toxin A and Toxin B which is coded by TcdA and TcdB which is responsible for mucosal injury and Inflammatory patches also there is cell water secretion causing watery diarrhea.
- The damaged and inflamed patches results in yellow white plaques or Pseudomembranous colonic mucosa which is covering erythematous colonic mucosa.

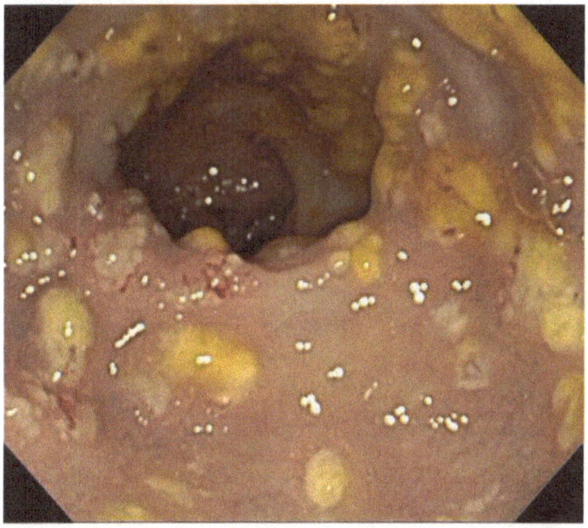

Source: Wikipedia; Author: Samir; License: Creative Commons Attribution 3.0 Unported license

- If the colonic injury is severe then it can lead to complications like Toxic megacolon, adynamic ileus, peritonitis, intestinal perforation.
- Diagnosis can be made by clostridium difficile exotoxin in stool via ELISA and colonoscopy for Pseudomembranous colitis.

37. 33 years old comes with complain of watery diarrhea and lower abdominal pain for the last 3 days. He has a history of pneumoniae for which he was hospitalized 2 weeks ago, during his hospitalisation he was given various antibiotics. Upon conducting her gram smear gram-positive purple colored rod shaped bacteria were seen. Which of the following is selective and differentiating culture for this organism?

A. Wilson and Blair Bismuth sulphite agar
B. Thayer Martin agar
C. Chocolate agar
D. Cycloserine-cefoxitin fructose agar

Answer: D. Cycloserine-cefoxitin fructose agar

Solution

- Clostridium difficile is purple color gram-positive rod shaped organism which produces Toxin A and Toxin B.
- These toxins are known to cause watery diarrhea and Pseudomembranous colon.

- In fulminant cases there can be complications like intestinal perforation, peritonitis, Toxic megacolon, Adynamic ileus.
- **Treatment for Clostridium Difficile:**
    1. **Mild/moderate disease**–Oral Metronidazole.
    2. **Severe cases**–Oral Vancomycin.
    3. **Fulminant cases**–Oral Vancomycin + IV Metronidazole.

38. 26 years old male was brought to Emergency room around 9:00 AM when his family found him unresponsive and didn't wake up from sleep. When he was examined patient was found to be dead. Family gives history of him going for a country side camping with his friends 2 days ago. They had locally processed pork for breakfast and exactly 6 hours after having breakfast he started having abdominal pain and diarrhea which later transformed into bloody diarrhea. Because of which he had to return home from camping next day. Instead of visiting hospital he decided to take NSAID along with ampicillin and have rest.

When autopsy was performed his abdomen was found to be distended along with 500 mL straw colored fluid in peritoneum. Microscopic examination of intestine revealed presence of necrosis. Along with gram smear showing gram-positive 'box car' appearance.Which of the following is NOT correct regarding organism causing patient's death?

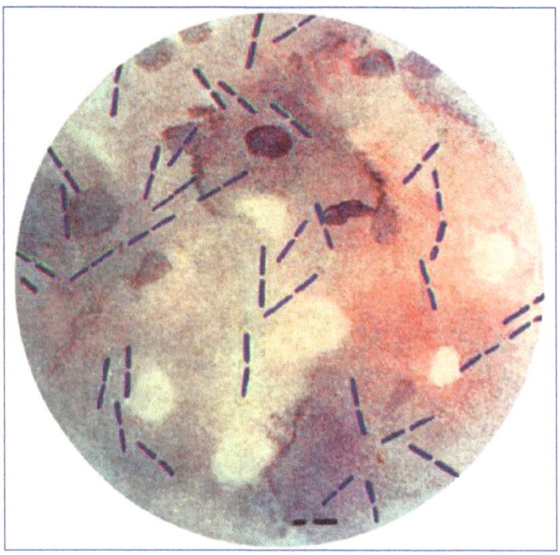

Box car appearance of gram-positive Clostridium perfringens

A. It can grow upto 45°C
B. It is reverse CAMP test positive
C. Target hemolysis is seen on blood agar
D. Stormy fermentation on litmus milk
E. It produces Toxin A and Toxin B

Answer: E. It produces Toxin A and Toxin B

Solution

- Clostridium perfringens is gram-positive purple colored rod shaped organism which is characteristically described as having box car shaped appearance.

- On blood agar it produces 'Target hemolysis' and is positive for reverse CAMP test.

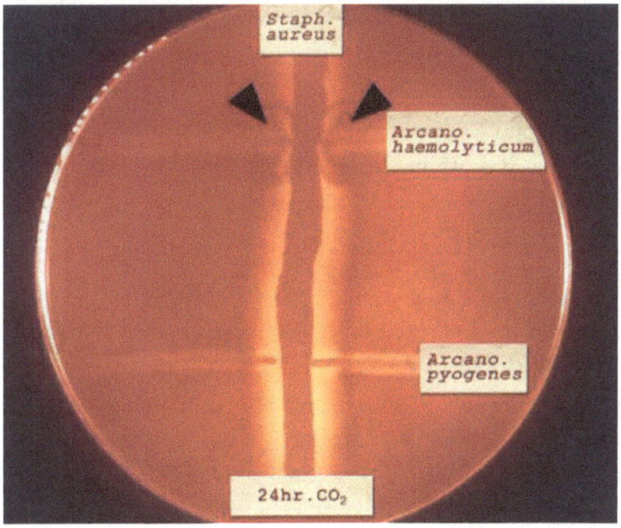

Reverse CAMP test

Target hemolysis on blood agar

- Clostridium perfringens causes stormy fermentation in litmus milk medium. As lactose in milk gets fermented into acid and gas. Acid coagulate milk protein casein into acid clot and along with gas production it shows stormy fermentation.
- Clostridium perfringens produces 12 histolytic toxins.

  There are 4 major toxins:

  1. Alpha (α) toxin (Most important)
  2. Beta (β) toxin
  3. Epsilon (ε) toxin
  4. Iota (ι) toxin
- These toxins are dermonecrotic and homolytic (hot and cold type) in nature.
- Test used to check presence of alpha toxin is 'Nagler's reaction'.

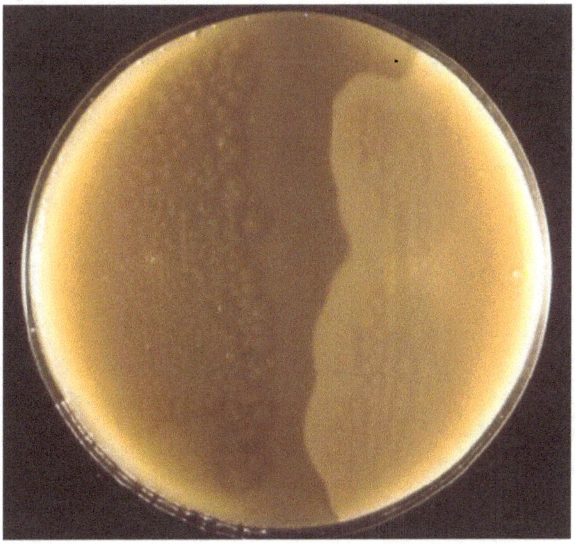

- Alpha toxin plays most important role in necrosis of tissue since it produces 'lecithenase', causes aggregation of platelet and intravascular hemolysis.
- The given case is that of pigbel or necrotising enteritis which is caused by 'type C clostridium perfringens'. It produces heat resistant spores.
- Generally found in pork meat.
- **Symptoms:** Bloody diarrhea, Abdominal pain.
- **Diagnosis:** Stool culture.
- **Treatment:** Parenteral penicillin + Metronidazole.

39. 32 years old female develops a shock state 12 hours after radical cystectomy with ileal conduit reconstruction. Her condition continued to deteriorate for next 5 hours and was finally decided to be transferred to Intensive Care Unit.

As soon as she was transferred to ICU hemorrhagic skin lesion appeared on her skin as given below in image. Suspecting it to be necrotising fasciitis emergency fasciotomy was performed along with multiple antibiotics, hyperbaric oxygen therapy. Culture of specimen retrieved from fasciotomy was performed and results are shown in images given below:

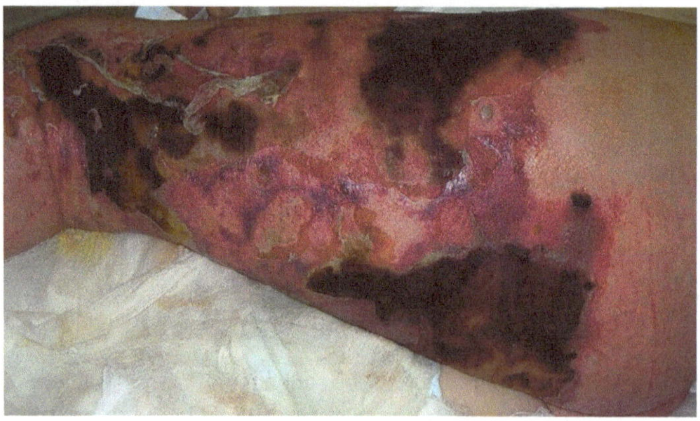

Necrotising fasciitis

Source: Late diagnosed necrotizing fasciitis as a cause of multiorgan dysfunction syndrome: A case report. Cases Journal 2008, 1:125. doi:10.1186/1757-1626-1-125, Author: Piotr Smuszkiewicz, Iwona Trojanowska and Hanna Tomczak; License: Creative Commons Attribution 3.0 Unported license

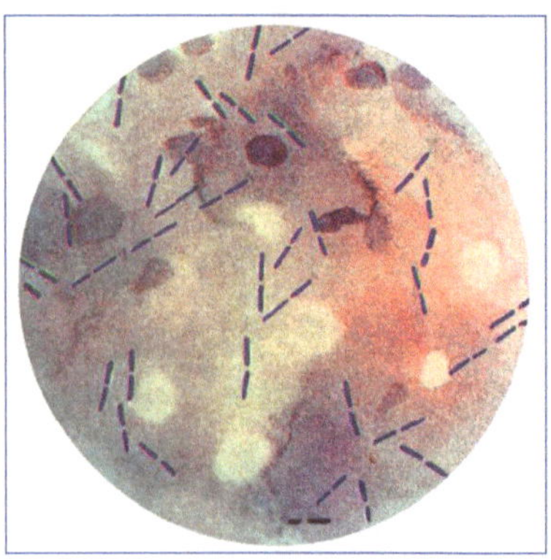

Gram smear

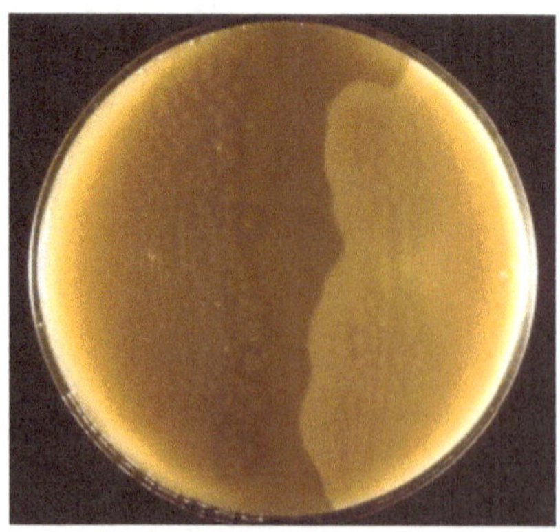

Nagler reaction showing presence of alpha toxin

Which of the following is correct regarding pathogenic organism?

A. One of the characteristic features of this organism is its ability to grow at 45°C

B. It has tennis racquet appearance

C. It produces round, convex, umbonate colonies in blood agar

D. It manifests swarming or Diene's phenomenon on blood agar

E. Its selective and differentiating medium is Thayer-Martin media

Answer: A. One of the characteristic features of this organism is its ability to grow at 45°C

Solution

- In the given case patient developed septic shock after radical cystectomy with ileal conduit reconstruction.
- It is most likely that ileum served as a source of infection.
- Clostridium are generally soil saprophytes.
- In GI flora there are 3 types of clostridium, i.e., Clostridium perfringens, Clostridium tetani, Clostridium ramosum.
- Clostridium perfringens produces alpha toxin which is most important for dermonecrosis also positive Nagler reaction proofs the existence of alpha toxin.This toxin is mainly responsible for necrotic fasciitis in the patient as given in image.
- Treatment for necrotising fasciitis and myonecrosis caused by Clostridium perfringens is surgical debridement, hyperbaric oxygen. Parenteral antibiotics-Penicillin + Clindamycin.
- On gram smear Clostridium perfringens appears as purple color along with box car appearance.
- On blood agar Clostridium perfringens has Target hemolysis.
- **For culture medium should have 2 characteristics:**
  1. Low redox potential.
  2. Anaerobiosing.
- **Example of cultivation medium are:**
  1. McIntosh and Fildes' anaerobic jar.
  2. Anaerobic gas pack.
  3. Robertson's Cooked Meat (RCM) medium.
- RCM contains pieces of fat-free minced cooked meat of ox heart and nutrient broth.
- If meat in RCM jar turns black then clostridium is proteolytic in nature.
- If meat turns pink then meat is saccharolytic in nature.
- Clostridium that are saccharolytic are Clostridium perfringens, Clostridium difficile, Clostridium novyi, Clostridium septicum.
- Clostridium that are proteolytic are Clostridium histolyticum, Clostridium sporogens, Clostridium bifermentous.

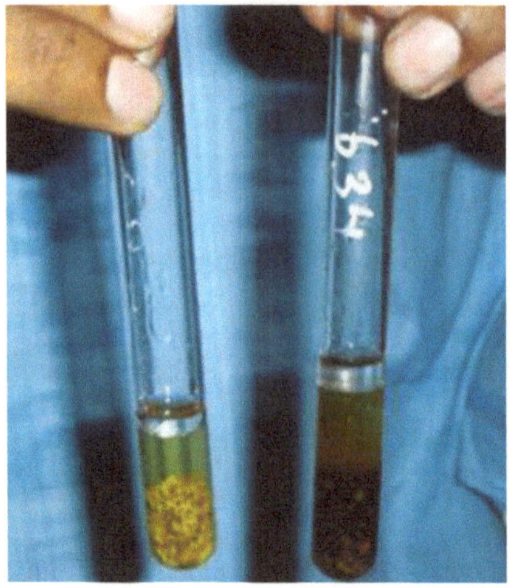

Source: Wikipedia; Author: Netha Hussain;

- Selective media for Clostridium perfringens can be Blood agar with Neomycin/Polymyxin.
- Media that can be used is enzyme based Pre Reduced Anaerobically Sterilised PRAS media.

40. In a district hospital 38 students of same school have been diagnosed with food poisoning in the last 2 days, coming with complain of abdominal pain and watery diarrhea. Upon conducting gram smear purple color gram-positive bacteria having 'box car appearance' was found, also PCR for 'CPE' gene came to be positive. Later doctor confirms that the causative organism is Clostridium perfringens. Medical officer of that district decides to conduct screening of food for Clostridium perfringens in school's canteen.

Which of the following media would be best for culture?

A. Thayer-Martin media
B. PRAS media
C. Chocolate media
D. CLED agar

Answer: B. PRAS media

Solution

- For culture of clostridium there are 2 necessary requirements:
  1. Low redox potential.
  2. Anaerobiosing.
- PRAS is enzyme based Pre Reduced Anaerobically Sterilised media.

41. 4 days old term neonate was brought to primary health care facility in rural area with complain of sudden inability to breastfeed, excessive crying and stiffening of body when touched. On admission there was autonomic dysfunction along with respiratory distress. Pediatrician conduct blood culture. On gram smear there was purple color gram-positive bacteria with drum stick or tennis racquet appearance as given below in image. On blood agar there is colonies formation in swarming layer over medium. Which of the following is used as culture media?

A. PRAS media
B. Wilson and Blair Bismuth sulphite
C. Mouse bioassay

Answer: C. Mouse bioassay

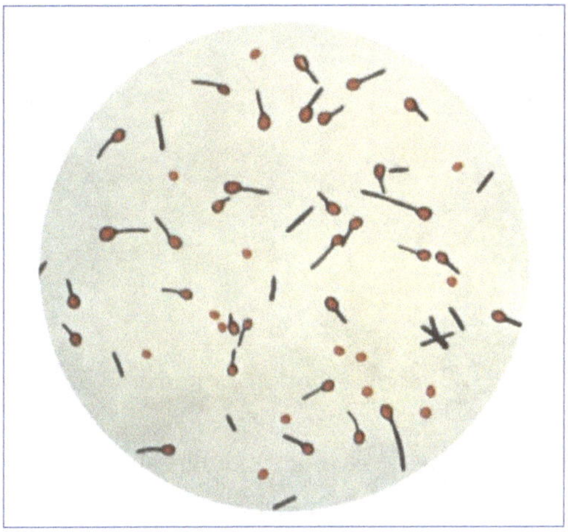

Gram smear showing Clostridium tetani

Solution

- Infant is suffering from 'Neonatal tetanus' which is generally seen in places of poor health facilities.
- Most probable source of infection is most likely to be cutting umbilical stump by non-sterilised instruments.
- In neonatal tetani child is born with normal ability to suck but between 3rd and 28th day child loses ability to suck and breastfeed becomes rigid and have spasms. This is due to toxin 'tetanospasmin' which causes presynaptic inhibition of release of inhibitory neurotoxin like GABA and glycine resulting in uncontrolled stimulation of motor neuron causing rigidity and spasm.
- Tetanospasmin cleaves synaptobrevin (VAMP) which is responsible for fusion of vesicles.
- Its primary site of action is ventral neuron of spinal cord and motor neuclei of Cranial Nerve.
- Culture used for Clostridium tetani is Mouse bioassay.

42. 20 years old male presents with generalised body stiffness, breathing difficulty and inability to swallow along with slurred speech. Patient is daily wage labour construction worker. He gives history of being injured by long nail in his foot around 15 days back. Upon examining wound is deep and dirty. No antiseptic or dressing was done for the injury. Doctor conducts a blood culture which showed purple colored gram-positive bacilli which had tennis racquet shaped or drum stick appearance. Which of the following test image given below would NOT be positive for this pathogenic bacteria? (Multiple answers can be correct).

A. 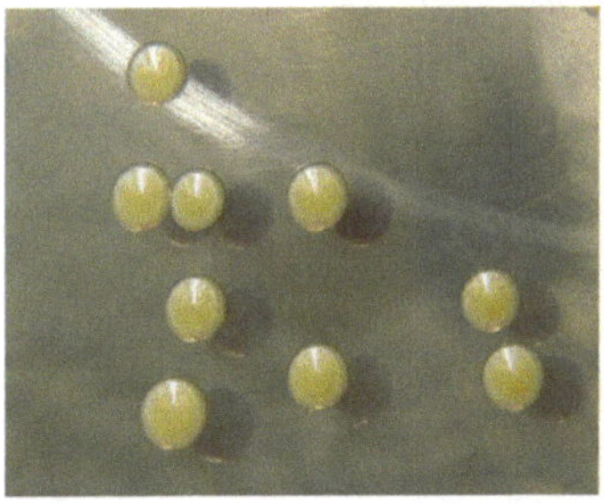

B. 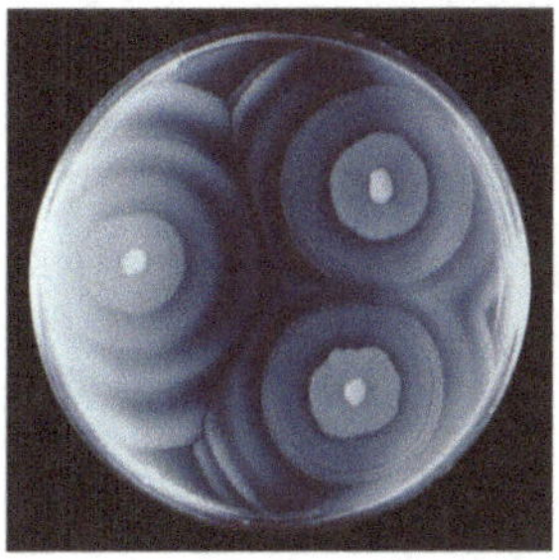

C. 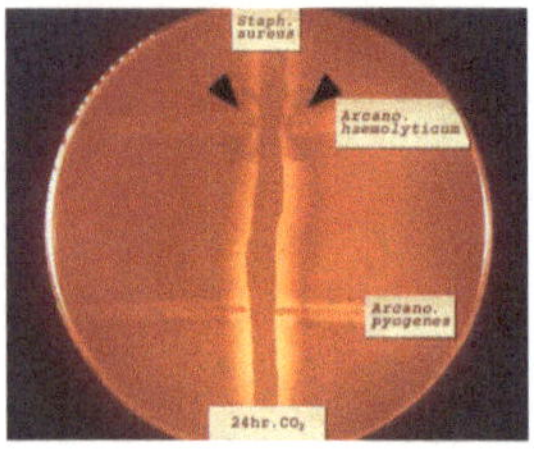

D. 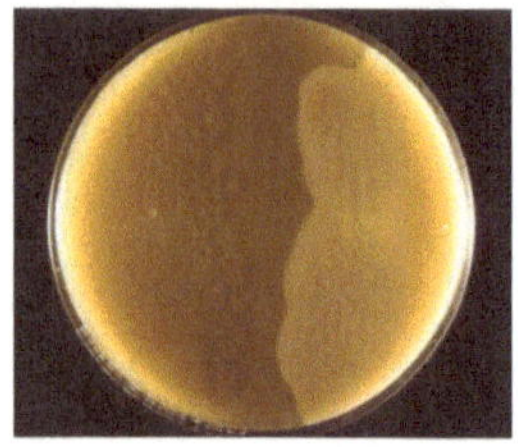

Answer: A, B, C and D

Solution

- Option A given image is that of Staphyloxanthin seen in case of Staphylococcus aureus when grown on nutrient agar.
- Option B given image is that of proteus which exhibits swarming as shown in image.
- Option C given image is that of clostridium perfringens manifest reverse CAMP test.
- Option D given image is that of Clostridium perfringens manifest Nagler's reaction.
- Test that are positive for Clostridium tetani are Gelatin stab test showing fir tree appearance.

Gelatin stab test and different appearances	
Organism	***Shape***
Clostridium tetani	Fir tree appearance
Bacillus anthracis	Inverted fir tree appearance
Vibrio cholera	Napiform and Infundibuliform

43. 21-year-old male comes with primary complain of painless raised lesion over his right hand along with chills and fever for last 3 days. Lesion is of 4 cm ulcerative in nature, raised and surrounded by edema as given in image below.

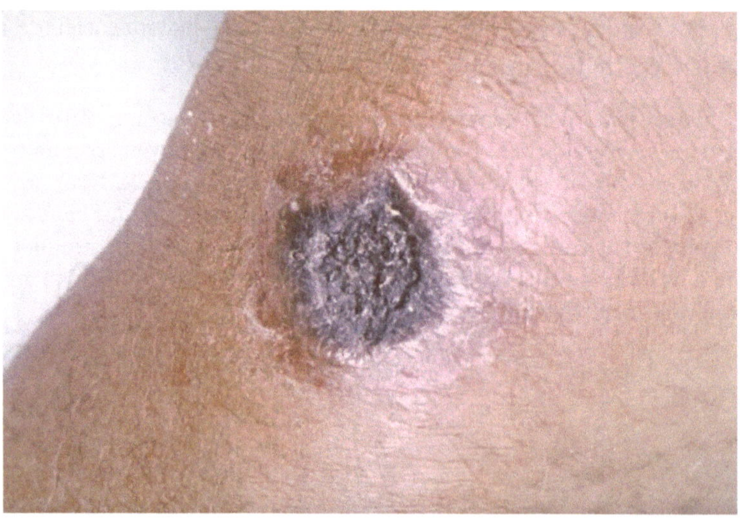

Patient has recently started working at butcher shop. Doctor conduct culture of lesion scrapings. Which of the following is NOT correct regarding culture of pathogenic organism?

A. On nutrient agar there is Medusa head appearance

B. Selective media is PLET

C. It manifests McFadyean Reaction

D. It shows string of pearl appearance when grown on media

E. Gelatin stab culture shows fir tree appearance

Answer: E. Gelatin stab culture shows fir tree appearance

Solution

- Patient is suffering from cutaneous bacillus anthracis infection.
- Bacillus anthracis is found naturally in soil.
- Its reservoir is grass eating animals.
- Infective form – spores.
- Compare cutaneous of bacillus, mycoplasma buruli ulcer, ecthyema gangrenous of pseudomonas and clostridium perfringens necrotising fasciitis which is also caused by strep Gp. A, clostridium perfringens, Klebsiella, E coli, staphylococcus aureus.

Note:

- The bacterias causing necrotising fasciitis are called "flesh eating bacterium" and some of the examples are:
  1. Group A Streptococcus (Most common).
  2. Clostridium perfringens.
  3. E. coli.
  4. Staphylococcus.
  5. Klebsiella.
  6. Aeromonas hydrophilia.
- Bacillus anthracis is gram-positive purple colored rod shaped bacteria that have 'Bamboo stick arrangement'.

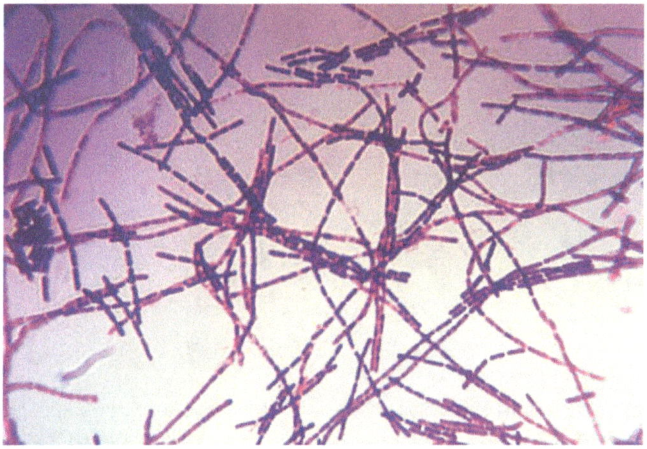

Bacillus anthracis gram smear showing Bamboo shaped appearance

- **Biochemical reactions of Bacillus anthracis:**
  1. Catalase positive.
  2. Oxidase positive.
  3. Ferment sugar.
  4. Gelatin stab culture–Inverted fir tree appearance.
  5. On nutrient agar there frosted glass appearance or Medusa head appearance.

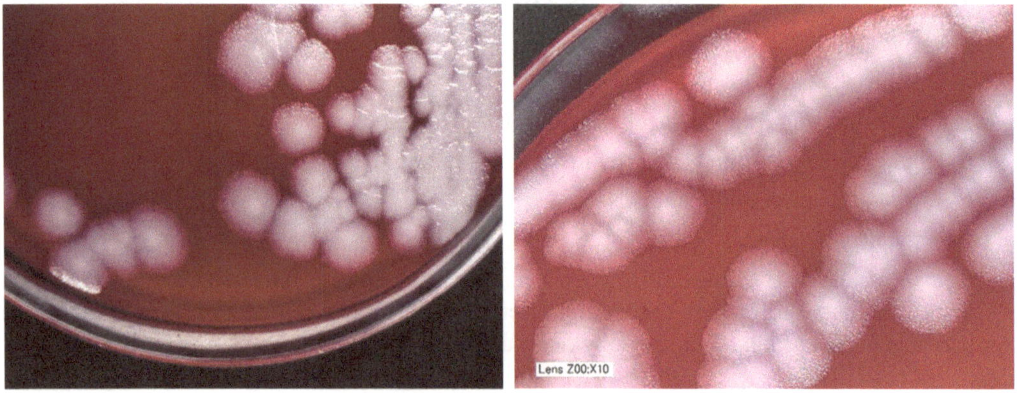

Bacillus anthracis on nutrient agar manifest 'Medusa head appearance or frosted glass appearance'

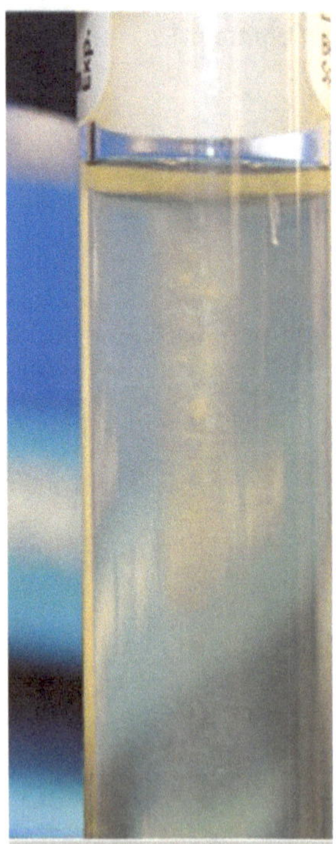

Gelatin stab culture of Bacillus anthracis showing inverted fir tree appearance

Source: File:OSC Microbio 09 02 listumbrel.jpg Author: CNX Open Stax; Creative Commons Attribution-ShareAlike 4.0 International license

6. Bacillus anthracis when grown on medium shows 'String of pearl reaction'.

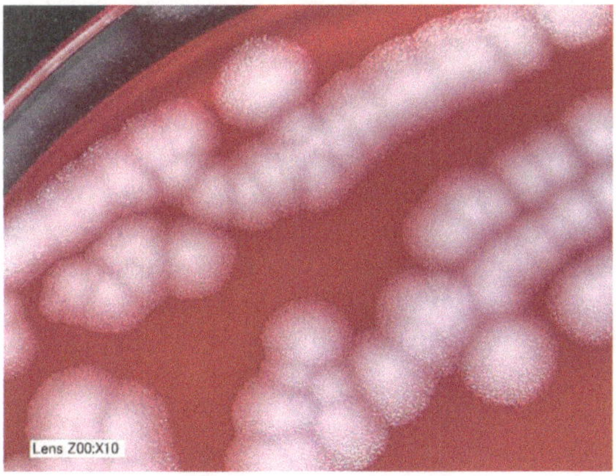

String of pearl reaction

7. Bacillus manifests 'McFadyean Reaction'. McFadyean Reaction is when Bacillus anthracis is grown on 'polychrome methylene blue' bacteria takes blue color and capsule around looks pinkish or amorphous material.

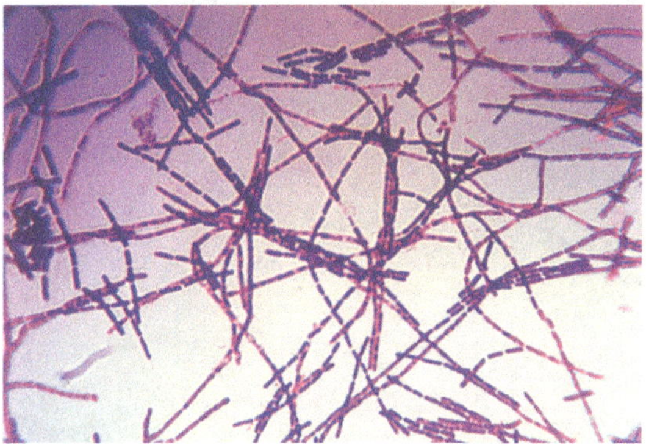

McFadyean reaction

8. Selective media–PLET media, contains Polymyxin, Lysozyme, EDTA, Tetra acetic acid contains EDTA.

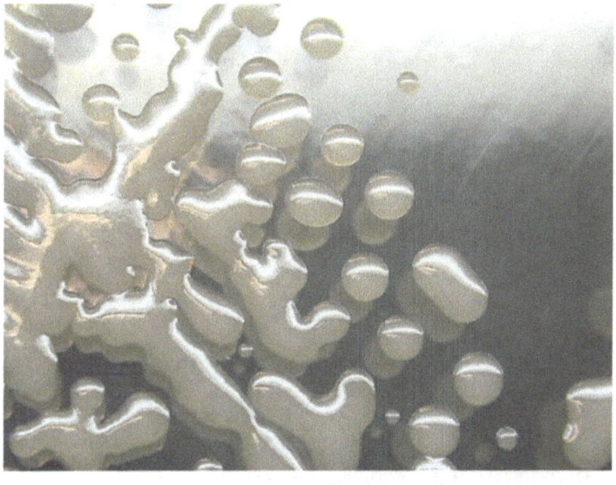

PLET media

- Generally Bacillus anthracis spread from domestic animals spores present in fluid released from animals is responsible for spread of infection.
- Spores are not formed in human so can't be seen in specimen.

44. 25 years old male presents with complain of abdominal pain, bloody diarrhea, nausea, fever and malaise for the last 3 days. Man belongs from a rural tribal community 3 days back, he butchered his own goat with his bare hands and had its meat for lunch. Doctor conducts and sends blood and stool specimen for results revealed presence of purple colour gram-positive bacteria that had bamboo sticks appearance. Also Gelatin stab test showed fir tree appearance. On nutrient agar there is frosted glass appearance or Medusa head appearance along with string of pearl reaction. Also test came out positive for McFadyean reaction. What should be next step in management?

A. Penicillin
B. Ampicillin
C. Ciprofloxacin + doxycycline
D. Amoxicillin

Answer: C. Ciprofloxacin + doxycycline

45. 23 years old male comes with complain of abdominal pain, vomiting, nausea, watery diarrhea for the last 6 hours after he had fried rice for breakfast in his college canteen. Upon conducting culture of his stool sample following finding were observed.

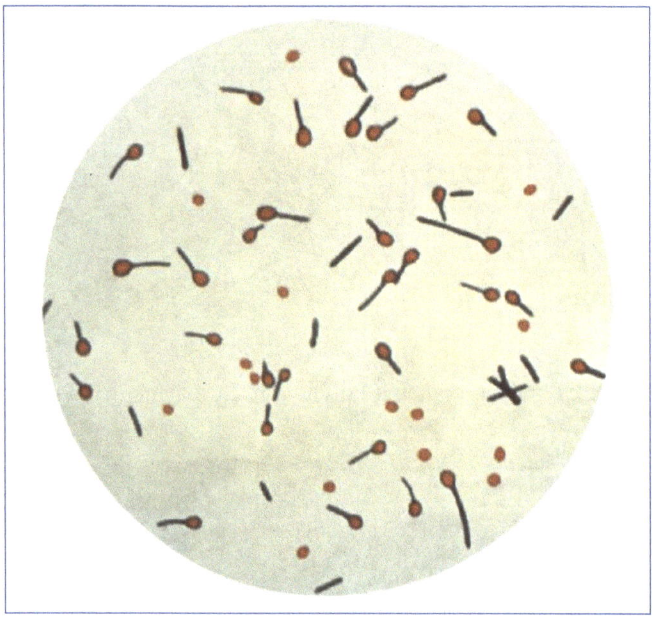

Gram smear

Name the causative organism and whether it is capsulated or not?

A. Bacillus cereus; non capsulated
B. Bacillus cereus; capsulated
C. Proteus, capsulated
D. Clostridium tetani, non capsulated

Answer: D. Clostridium tetani, non capsulated

Solution

- Given case is of food poisoning and image given is of Hemolytic swarming growth on blood agar.
- Gram-positive organism showing swarming growth on blood agar are Clostridium tetani, Bacillus cereus.
- Gram-negative organism showing swarming growth on blood agar are Proteus mirabilis, Proteus vulgaris.

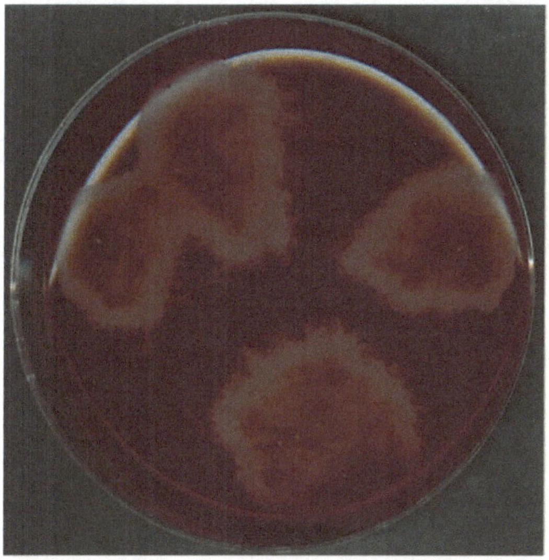

Bacillus cereus shows swarming on blood agar (Hemolytic)

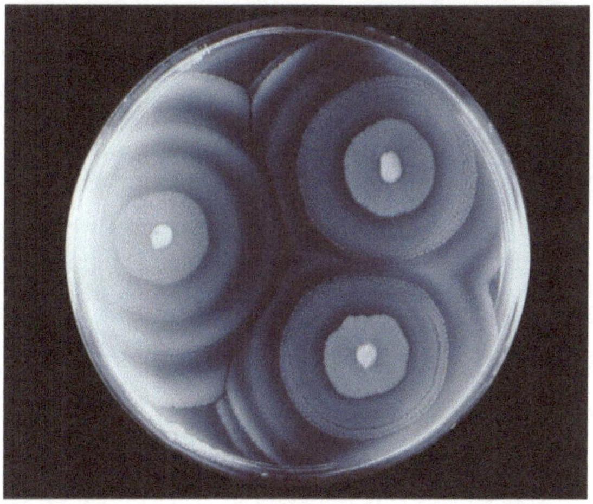

Proteus showing swarming growth on blood agar

- Bacillus cereus is gram-positive bacilli but on Gram stain it appears to be pink because its cell wall is surrounded by a lot of complex structure so Gram stain can't reach up to cell wall.
- Selective media–MYPA Mannitol egg Yolk Phenol red Polymyxin Agar.

46. 32 years old man presented with complain of dyspnea, sore throat, muscle ache for last 7 days. He has recently started domesticating sheeps. He has no personal or family history of COPD or other respiratory pathology. While examining the patient his oxygen was assessed by oximeter which came out to be 92%, his heart rate was increased, Blood pressure was 165/90. Doctor conducts X-ray imaging which showed presence of pneumonia. Patient's blood was sent for culture which showed purple colored gram-positive bacteria which had bamboo stick appearance. It was also positive for McFadyean's reaction. On blood agar there was Medusa head appearance or frosted glass appearance along with string of pearl reaction. Gelatin stab test showed inverted fir tree appearance. What is the mechanism of toxin produced by causative organism?

A. Toxins act by inhibition of Mitogen-activated protein kinase (MAPK) pathway causing cell death

B. Toxins act by inhibiting reuptake of inhibitory neurotransmitters at nerve endings

C. Toxin inhibits protein synthesis by ADP ribosylation

Answer: A. Toxins act by inhibition of Mitogen-activated protein kinase (MAPK) pathway causing cell death

Solution

- Bacillus anthracis produces anthrax toxin which have 3 factors:
  1. Edema factor.
  2. Lethal factor.
  3. Protective factor.
- These factors finally lead into inhibition of MAPK's.
- In epidic region of Bacillus anthracis Anthrax vaccine is given which is 5 dose regimen.
- For post exposure prophylaxis we give Doxycycline or Ciprofloxacin/Levofloxacin or Amoxicillin for 60 days.

47. 6 years old female brought in with complain of 2 cm ulcerous lesion with undetermined margins along with necrosis present on dorsal aspect of left arm superior to the elbow joint.

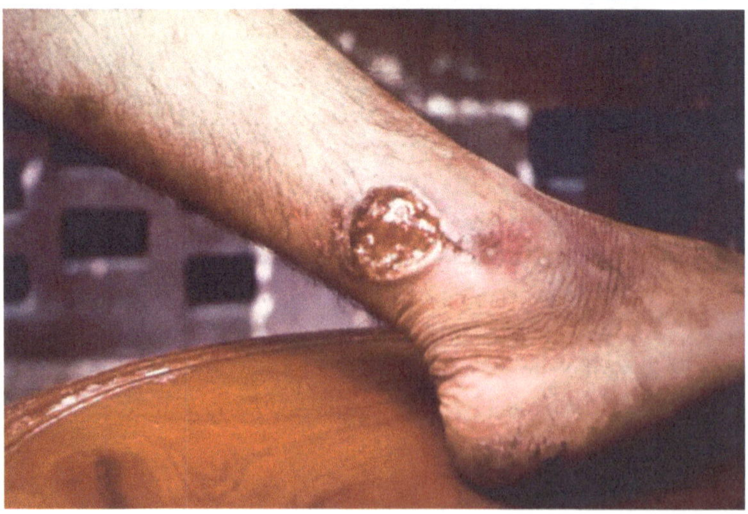

Patient belongs from rural area with low socioeconomic status. Patient has incomplete vaccination status. Considering it to be case of mycobacterium ulcerans doctor send the lesion scrapings for Ziehl-Neelsen stain/ZN staining or Kinyoun stain which came out to be positive. Which of the following is used for culture of organism?

A. Löwenstein-Jensen medium or LJ media
B. Thayer-Martin media
C. PRAS
D. Cetrimide agar media

Answer: A. Löwenstein-Jensen medium or LJ media

Solution

- The given case is of buruli ulcer caused by Mycobacterium ulcerans.
- Child vaccine immunisation is incomplete hence she is at high risk of being infected by Mycobacterium, in this case Mycobacterium ulcerans.
- Mycobacterium is Acid Fast Bacilli (AFB) which is stained red in Ziehl-Neelsen stain or ZN stain.
- Mycobacterium is also stained red by Kinyoun stain.

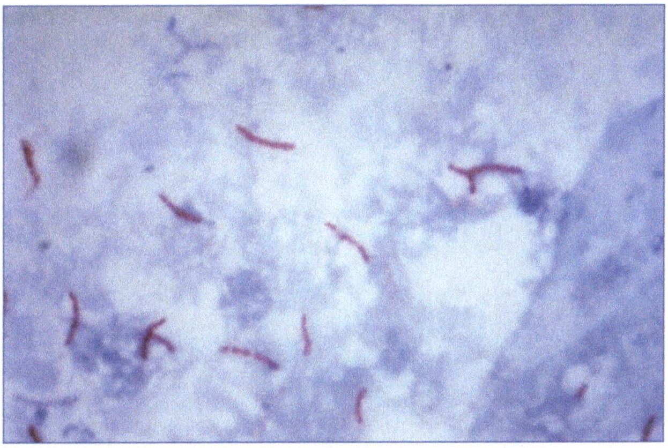

Ziehl-Neelsen stain

- Culture media for Mycobacterium is Lowenstein Jensen media or LJ media.

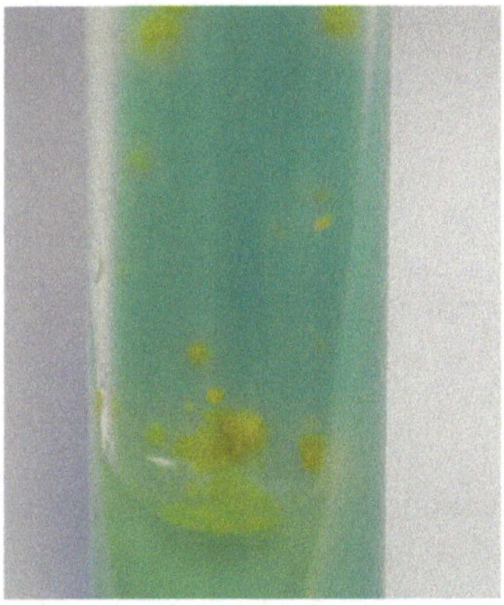

Lowenstein Jensen media

Source: Wikipedia; Author: Nathan Reading from Halesowen, UK;

- Mycobacterium ulcerans causes erosion of skin and underline tissue has cotton-wool like appearance.
- Mycobacterium ulcerans is caused by water borne skin pathogen, atypical Mycobacterium.
- It is mostly seen in West Africa and Australia.
- Bruli begins as firm painless subcutaneous nodule.
- Ulcerans begins weeks after nodule as skin starts to erode away leaving behind undermined edges and necrosis can be beyond the margin in subcutaneous tissue hence actual lesion is much larger than it seems.
- Complications nerve and vessel damage.
- **Treatment:** Oral Rifampicin + IV Streptomycin for 8 weeks.

48. 22 years old male comes with complain of dyspnea, cough for last 10 days along with chronic mild right sided flank pain that radiates through buttock to the left thigh along with fever and malaise for the last 7 days. He has a recent history of getting infected with COVID-19 one month ago and he remained on steroids for 10 days. On clinical examination it was noticed that patient had 'Antalgic gait' ipsilateral hip was in flexed and externally rotated position at rest. On passive extension and internal rotation there was elicit pain. Also tender mass was palpable in iliac region along with swollen cervical lymph nodes and illiac lymph nodes.

Doctor conducts CT scan and sputum ZN staining which showed following findings.

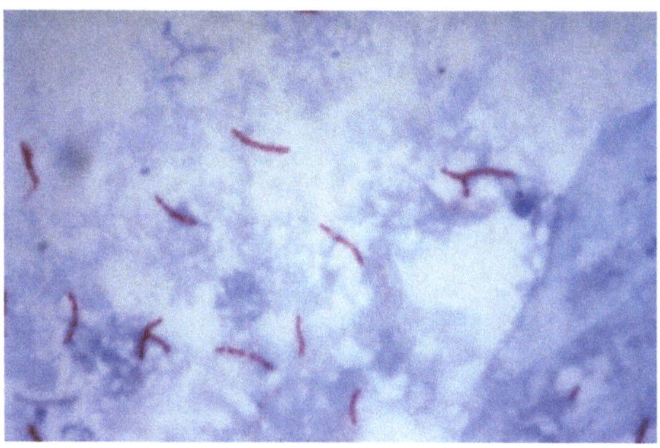

ZN stain showing Acid Fast Bacilli

Colonies that grew on solid media developed pigment in light and dark and took more than 7 days to develop in media.What is the most probable organism responsible for patients condition?

A. Mycobacterium scrofulaceum
B. Mycobacterium kansasii
C. Mycobacterium ulcerans
D. Mycobacterium fortuitum

Answer: A. Mycobacterium scrofulaceum

Solution

- According to Runyon classification Mycobacterium scrofulaceum comes under scotochromogenic mycobacteria.
- It is second most common cause for lymphadenitis caused by atypical Mycobacterium scrofulaceum is acid fast bacilli which stain red in ZN media and Kinyoun stain and can't be stained by Gram staining technique cause of high lipid content.

Runyon Classification

Group	*Defining characteristics*	*Examples*
Photochromogens	Produce pigmentation only in light and takes more than 7 days to grow in solid media	M. kansasii, M. marinum, M. simiae, M. asciaticum
Scotochromogens	Produce pigmentation in light and dark, takes more than 7 days to grow in solid media	M. scrofulaceum, M. szulgai, M. gordonae
Non photochromogens	Do not produce pigmentation and takes more than 7 days to grow in solid media	MAC, M. ulcerans, M. xenopi
Rapid growers	Takes less than 7 days to grow	M. fortuitum, M. chelonei, M. smegmatis

49. 21 years old male comes with complain of fever and malaise along with lesion on dorsum of his right hand as shown below.

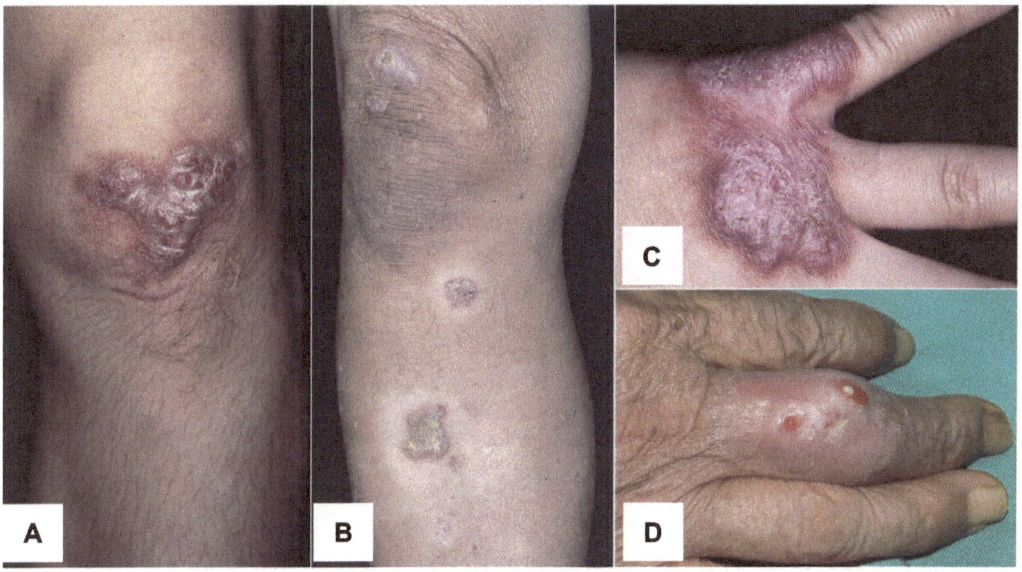

Patient is obese with BMI of 35 and has uncontrolled Diabetes for last 6 months. He is in compliant with his diabetic medication. He has family history of both his parents being diabetic and are on insulin for more than 20 years. Patient has recently started working at pet shop that also deals with selling of fish tanks and related aquarium fishes. Based on this doctor conducts lesion scrapings and send it for ZN staining and Kinyoun staining which showed red colour acid fast bacilli. Most likely causative mycobacterium belong to which Runyon's classification?

A. Photochromogenic
B. Scotochromogenic
C. Non photochromogenic
D. Rapid growers

Answer: A. Photochromogenic

Solution

- The given case described is that of 'Fish tank granuloma' or 'swimming pool granuloma'.
- It is caused by 'mycobacterium marinum' and generally spread by contact of infected water or fishes through minimal skin trauma.
- Incubation period is 2-3 weeks.
- At the site of lesion there can be itching or burning sensation.

50. 34 years old female comes with complain of mild fever and swelling and discharge at herniorrhaphy wound 5 days after hernioplasty surgery. On examination swelling is 2 cm × 2 cm in size, fluctuant and tender with defining borders. The discharge was sent for gram smear which showed gram-positive bacilli. On ZN staining, Kinyoun staining also in there is red colour Acid Fast Bacilli. On LJ media there were non chromogenic buff colored colonies were seen on day 5. Which of the following is causative organism?

A. Mycobacterium marinum
B. Mycobacterium kansasii
C. Mycobacterium fortuitum
D. MAC

Answer: C. Mycobacterium fortuitum

Solution

- Atypical Myobacterium Rapid growers are mainly responsible for skin and soft tissue infection which can occur post trauma/surgery/injection abscess.

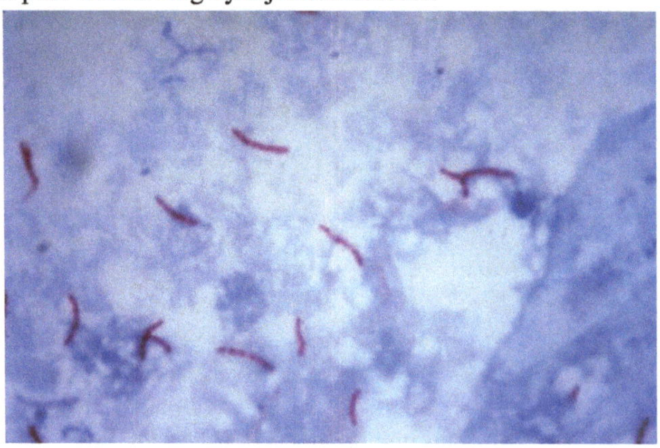

ZN stain showing red colour Acid Fast Bacilli

- Rhodamine auramine stain have Auramine 'O' and + Rhodamine 'B' binds to mycolic acid.

51. 11 months old infant is brought to emergency room with multiple complaints of fever and rash like lesion for the last 6 days and complain of seizures that occurred few hours before. Mother of infant told that fever was around 102°C and seizure lasted for around 1 minute in which infant's arms and legs were jerking and his eyes rolled up (only white sclera was visible), infant also micturated at that time. Birth of the child was uneventful through normal vaginal delivery at 37 weeks of gestation. There was no other significant history that was associated with infant since birth. Vaccination status of the infant was complete. There is no associated family for 2 generations with regard to any epileptic syndrome or seizure. Based on this consulting doctor sends the blood

for Complete Blood Count and also conducts Lumbar puncture. Complete Blood Count showed 25% Neutrophils and 50% Lymphocytes. For the lumbar puncture CSF was clear with increased amount of lymphocytes, Glucose was in normal range, i.e., >⅔rd of plasma glucose. Based on this doctor conducts a serological test for TORCHes which later came out to be positive for HHV-6. Which of the following is correct regarding this pathogenic organism?

A. Site of latency is at T-cell, B-cell, natural killer cell

B. It causes Roseola infantum/exanthema subitum

C. Primary infection or reactivation in immunocompromised may cause disseminated disease specially causing Pneumonia and encephalitis

D. Reactivation in immunocompromised causes herpes labialis

Answer: D. Reactivation in immunocompromised causes herpes labialis

Solution

- This is the case of Roseola infantum/exanthema subitum caused by HHV-6.
- **Mode of Transmission:** Mainly by saliva, genital secretions.
- **Site of latency:** T-cell, B-cell, natural killer cell.
- Reaction only seen in immunocompromised.
- **Clinical Presentation:**
  1. Fever.
  2. Rash.
  3. Seizure.
  4. Pneumonia.
- **Diagnosis:** Serology via PCR or NAAT's.
- **Treatment:** Ganciclovir.

52. 3 years old male child from Pakistan is brought to OPD with multiple complain of fever, headache and malaise related symptoms for the last 7 days, also child is experiencing neck rigidity and photophobia for the last 3 days. Birth of the child was uneventful via normal vaginal delivery at 37 weeks of gestation. Vaccine status of child is incomplete. Based on this consulting doctor send the blood for Complete Blood Count and conducted Lumbar puncture. The blood report was normal with no increase in WBC or neutrophils or lymphocytes. The CSF was clear with increased lymphocytes and glucose was more than ⅔rd of plasma glucose along with minimal increase in protein.

At this stage doctor send blood for serology testing for mumps, measles, rubella, herpes, flavivirus, polio, coxsackie, ECHO virus. All of them came to be negative except for polio IgM came out to be positive. At this stage your professor ask you which of the following is NOT true with regards to paralytic polio?

A. It belongs to Enterovirus C

B. Anti D antibody provides type specific immunity against VP-1 type of poliovirus

C. Larger muscle are affected more

D. Receptor for poliovirus is CD-155

E. Earliest change seen in case of poliovirus infection is Neurodegeneration of Nissl body/ chromatolysis

F. Blood remains positive for poliovirus 3 weeks after infection

Answer: F. Blood remains positive for poliovirus 3 weeks after infection

Solution

- This is the rare case of paralytic polio which is completely eradicated from most of countries of world except Pakistan and Afghanistan.
- Poliovirus comes under category of Enterovirus and it belongs to Enterovirus C.
- Picorna virus which is smallest RNA virus is classified into:
  1. Enterovirus
  2. Rhinovirus
- The most characteristic difference between Enterovirus and Rhinovirus is that Rhinovirus is acid labile while Enterovirus remains stable for pH 3-10.
- **Polio:** Gray.
- **Myelitis:** Spinal cord inflammation.
- Poliovirus that is part of Enterovirus C.
- Based on antigen on VP-1, VP-2, VP-3 protein there are 3 types of poliovirus:
  - *Type-1:* Most widespread.
  - *Type-2:* Most antigenic and easiest to eradicate.
  - *Type-3:* Most commonly associated with paralytic illness.
- **Mode of Transmission:** Feco-oral route, retrograde axonal transport.

Clinical Features:

- Initially there would be prodromal symptoms followed by paralytic symptoms.
- On the basis of paralytic symptoms there can be 2 types of polio:
  1. **Spinal polio:** Initially there would be symptoms related to aseptic meningitis like fever, neck rigidity, photophobia etc.
     - Later there would be muscle involvement causing asymetrical flaccid paralysis.
     - Bigger muscle are affected more.
  2. **Bulbar paralytic polio myelitis:** There is involvement of Cranial Nerve 9 and 10 with muscle of soft palate and pharynx getting affected leading to symptoms like pooling of secretion in mouth, dysphagia, nasal speech and dyspnea.

Diagnosis:

- By serology or by molecular methods like PCR and NAAT's.
- For the specimen:
  1. **Blood:** Remains positive for 3-5 days after infection.
  2. **Throat swab:** Positive for upto 3 weeks after infection.
  3. **Stool:** Positive for 12 weeks after infection.

Complications:

- Respiratory problems may occur due to involvement of diaphragm or related Cranial Nerve, i.e., C-3, C-4, C-5.
- Detrussor muscle involvement can cause urinary retention.
- **Treatment** is mainly supportive.

53. 33 years old male presented with complain of nausea, vomiting and abdominal pain for the last 5 days, he is also experiencing fever, malaise along with dyspnea for the last 3 days. Vomiting was non bilious, non projectile with no blood stain. His fever was 102°C. Patient works at dairy farm. He is diabetic for the last 10 years and is on Metformin and gliflozin.

Upon examining the patient it was noticed that he is having mild icterus, his pulse rate was 72, respiratory rate of 16, oximeter showed oxygen levels to be 90%, his BP is 165/95. His X-ray report shows presence of pneumoniae. Also his hepatic enzymes were deranged. Upon conducting gram smear for peripheral blood no pathogenic organism was seen. What is most likely cause for patient's condition?

A. Q fever caused by coxiella burnetii

B. Disseminatied tuberculosis caused by Mycobacterium

C. Bartonella infection

D. Hepatitis B

Answer: A. Q fever caused by Coxiella burnetii

Solution

- In the given clinical scenario is most likely to be a case of Q fever caused by Coxiella burnetii because of relative bradycardia and patient association with dairy farm and consumption of raw dairy products.
- Coxiella burnetii is Gram-negative coccobacilli, 'obligate intracellular organism'.
- **Reservoir:** Domestic animals like cow, sheep, goat.
- **Mode of Infection:** Raw milk, Inhalation of aerosol percutaneous handling of animal products.
- There are 2 stages of Q fever:
  1. Acute
  2. Chronic
- In acute stage there is fever, chills, myalgia. These symptoms resolve spontaneously.
- In 5% of cases there can be pneumomia and hepatitis.
- In chronic cases there is large nodular vegetation of heart valve.There is very characteristic Culture negative endocarditis.

Diagnosis:

- For acute stage by collecting blood sample and use special type of cell line, i.e., 'Shell vial culture'.
- In acute phase Q fever there is increase in IgM antibodies while in chronic stage there is increase in IgG antibodies.

Note:

- In certain infection particularly intracellular gram-negative organism we notice relative bradycardia that is heart rate of patient is lower than expected for a given body temperature (it is applied only when temperature is more than 102°C).

- Organisms manifesting relative bradycardia are Chlamydia, legionella, typhoid fever, mycoplasma and rickettsia.

54. 40 years old male comes with complain of night sweats, shortness of breath, swelling of feet and weight loss for last 4 days. He is also having mild fever, chills, malaise for the last few weeks. Patient works in a dairy farm and was diagnosed with HIV 1 year ago. Upon examining he had BP of 110/70 with pulse of 87 and oximeter showed 93% oxygen, there was presence of Janeway lesion, splinter hemorrhage, Osler's nodule (images given below).

Upon conducting cardiac examination there was normal looking chest, no thrill on palpation, no vigor of contractility. On auscultation there is normal S1 and S2 with aortic regurgitation murmur.

On ECG there is widening of PR interval, p mitrale, T Wave Inversion (TWI) Trans Esophageal ECHO showed intracardial mass on valve.

Blood culture was conducted twice and both time came out to be negative. Later blood culture was done on 'Shell vial culture' which came to be positive. Based on the observations which antibiotics should be considered for this patient?

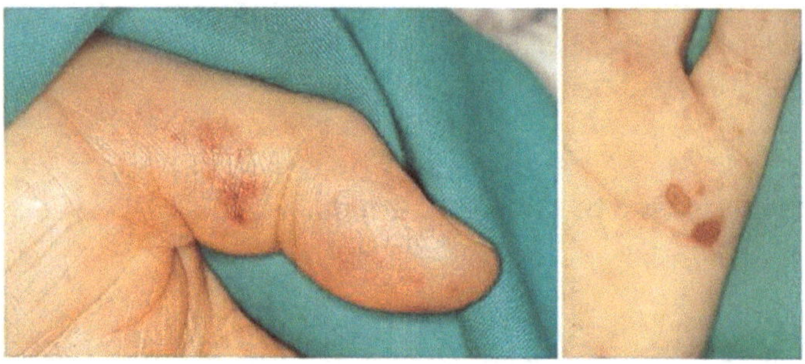

Osler's nodule

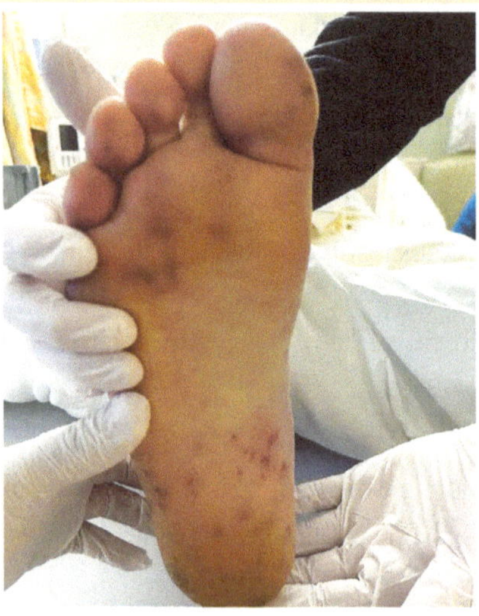

Janeway lesion

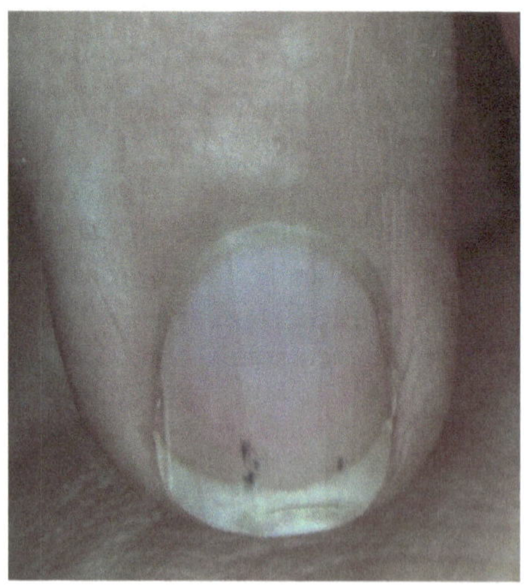

Splinter hemorrhage

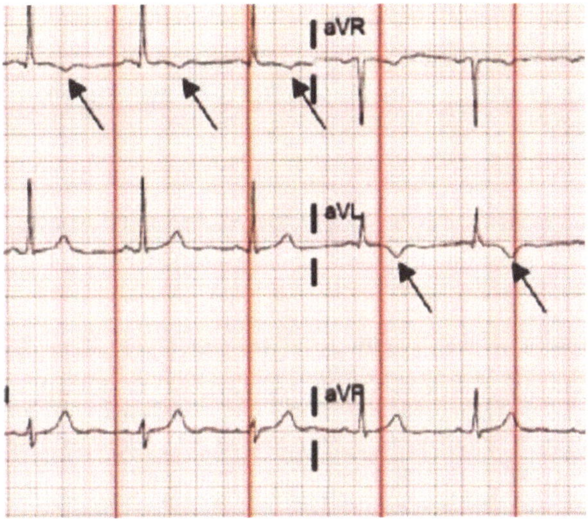

ECG showing T wave inversion

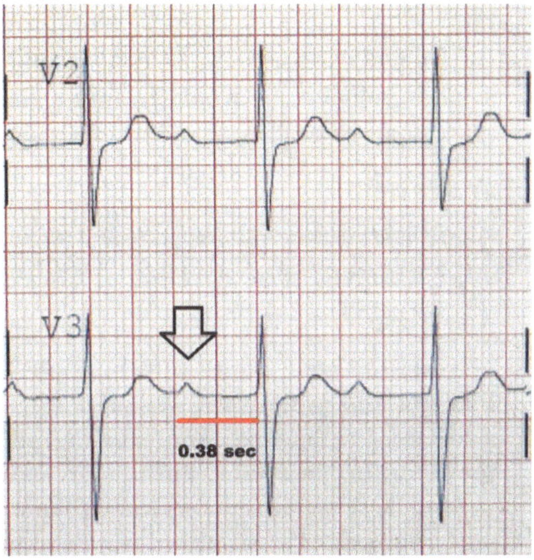

Increase PR interval

A. Doxycycline + Hydroxychloroquine/Rifampicin/Ciprofloxacin for 2-4 years

B. Doxycycline for 2-4 weeks

C. Ampicillin for 3 months

D. Penicillin for 3 months

Answer: A. Doxycycline + Hydroxychloroquine/Rifampicin/Ciprofloxacin for 2-4 years

Solution

- The given case is that of culture negative.
- Infective endocarditis caused by obligate intracellular Coxiella burnetii.
- Reservoir for Coxiella burnetii is domestic animals like cow, sheep and goat.
- Mode of infection for Coxiella burnetii is Consumption of raw milk, percutaneous inhalation of animal products and inhalation of aerosol etc.
- There are 2 stages of Q fever:
  1. Acute
  2. Chronic
- In acute phase of Coxiella burnetii there is fever, malaise and myalgia.
- 5% can also have hepatitis and pneumonia.
- Most common manifestation of Coxiella burnetii is 'Culture negative endocarditis'.
- **Risk factors for Q fever going into chronic stage are:**
  1. HIV infected individual.
  2. Chronic renal failure.
  3. Damaged or prosthetic heart valve.

Diagnosis:

- Culture in special type of cell line called 'Shell vial culture'.
- In serology there would be IgM antibodies present in acute phase of Coxiella burnetii, while in chronic stage there would be IgG antibodies.

Treatment:

- In acute phase with hepatitis and pneumonia the Drug of Choice is Doxycycline for 2-4 weeks.
- For chronic stage the Drug of Choice is Doxycycline + Hydroxychloroquine/Rifampicin/Ciprofloxacin for 2-4 years.

55. 23 years old male comes with multiple complain of neck swellings for the last 1 year, fever for 1 month and generalised weakness for 1 week. He is student of final year doctor of veterinary medicine. On detailed history he had single swelling present anteriorly not associated with any joint swelling, morning stiffness or tenderness in small joint. Later another 2 more swellings appeared in posterior cervical region. Upon examination 4 swellings were noticed in right posterior cervical region they were non tender, non erythematous, firm, non mobile with no sinus discharge. Largest one being 2 × 1 cm in size while other 3 were 1 × 1 cm in size. On conducting lymph node biopsy with Warthin-Starry (WS) staining there are clumps of pleomorphic Bacilli around endothelial cell. What is the causative organism responsible for patient's condition?

A. Coxiella burnetii
B. Mycobacterium scrofulaceum
C. MAC
D. Bartonella henselae

Answer: D. Bartonella henselae

Solution

- The given case is that of 'Cat Scratch disease' caused by Bartonella henselae.
- Bartonella henselae infection is associated with exposure to cat since patient is student of veterinary medicine it puts him in high risk of developing this pathology.
- **Mode of infection:** Cat bite or scratch or cat lick over skin abrasion.
- **Incubation period:** 3-10 days.
- Symptoms of Bartonella henselae in non HIV or healthy individuals are papule like lesion along with Ipsilateral lymphadenopathy.
- Generally resolves spontaneously.
- For diagnosis biopsy is done with 'Warthin Starry Silver Stain'.
- **Drug of choice:** Erythromycin or Doxycycline.

56. It was reported to you in your hospital that 35-40 prisoners imprisoned in the same jail have fallen ill for the last 1 month while one of them recently have ended up in state of coma. They all are reported to have similar symptoms like fever, night sweats, myalgia along with rashes on trunk (shown below). Upon further inquiring it was found that some of them were having delirium and stupor related symptoms. Based on this description consultant in your hospital asked you that what would be the most likely outcome if we perform Neil Mooser reaction for this patient?

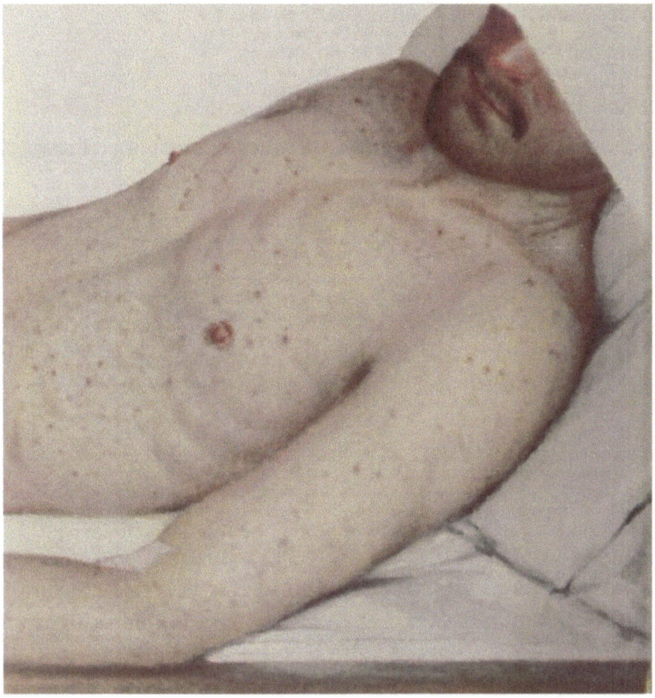

Source: Wikipedia; Lehrbuch der Infektionskrankheiten fur Arzte und studierende by Jochmann, Georg. Publication date 1914 Author:Georg Jochmann; License: sCreative Commons Attribution 4.0 international license

A. Scrotal necrosis

B. Fever only

C. Inflammation of testis (Testis can't be pushed into abdomen)

D. Causative organism is Coxiella burnetii hence Neil Mooser test should not be performed in these patients

Answer: B. Fever only

Solution

- The given case is most likely of Epidemic typhus caused by Ricketssia prowazekii.
- Ricketssia mainly causes 2 types of disease:
  1. **Typhous group:** CNS symptoms are dominant.
  2. **Spotted fever group:** Rash dominant.
- Epidemic typhus or jail fever is caused by Ricketssia prowazekii.
- **Vector:** Body louse.
- **Reservoir:** Man and flying squirrels.
- **Mode of infection:** Mucous membrane or skin break exposure to louse feces.
- **Clinical features:** Fever + rash starting from trunk, myalgia, stupor, delirium or coma.
- Epidemic typhus is called Jail fever because it is seen generally where there is overcrowding and low living standards.

- **Diagnosis** done by species specific antibodies.
- **Treatment: Drug of Choice** -> Doxycycline.

Neil Mooser or Tunica Test:

- In this test blood sample is collected from the patient and inoculated intraperitoneally in male guinea pig.

Neil Mooser or Tunica Reaction

Rickettsia species	*Result*
Rickettsia rickettsii	Scrotal necrosis (Strongly positive test)
Rickettsia typhi, Rickettsia akari, Rickettsia conorii	Inflammation (Testis can't be pushed into abdomen) (Positive test)
Rickettsia prowazekii	Fever only (Negative test)
Scrub typhus	No response seen in guinea pig (Negative test)

57. 60 years old male Japanese in origin comes to OPD with complain of fever, loss of appetite and headache for last 6 days along with swelling in posterior cervical region in last 2 days. He gives history of returning from Japan 8 days ago. While he was in Japan he used to visit Mountain to collect edible plant. He denies any sort of animal contact. On physical examination he had purple colored non pruritic eruption observed on face, extremities and trunk as shown in image and eschar in left upper limb as given in image below.

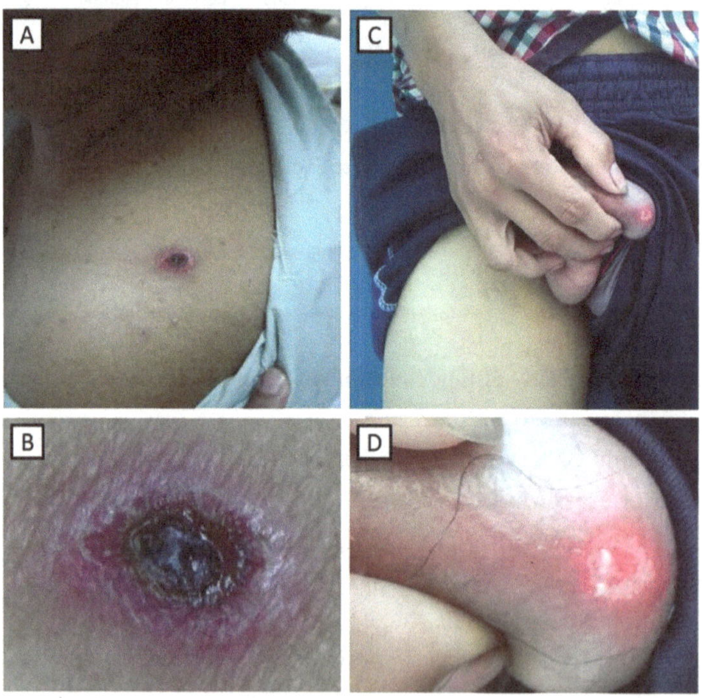

Source: Wikipedia; Use of eschar swabbing for the molecular diagnosis and genotyping of Orientia tsutsugamushi causing scrub typhus in Quang Nam province, Vietnam. PLoS Negl Trop Dis. 2017 Feb 27;11(2): e0005397. doi: 10.1371/journal.pntd.0005397
Author: Le Viet N, Laroche M, Thi Pham HL, Viet NL, Mediannikov O, Raoult D, Parola P; License: Creative Commons Attribution-ShareAlike 4.0 International license

Your senior consultant is highly suspicious it to be the case of Scrub typhus also known as chiggerosis. Your senior consultant ask you to name Heterophile antigen between Proteus and Scrub typhus, also which antibiotics would be contraindicated in this patient?

A. Ox-K of Proteus mirabilis and sulphonamide

B. Ox-2 of Proteus vulgaris and fluoroquinolones

C. Ox-19 of Proteus vulgaris and penicillin

D. Ox-K of Proteus mirabilis and penicillin

Answer: A. Ox-K Proteus mirabilis and sulphonamide

Solution

- The given case is of Scrub typhus caused by 'orientia tsutsugamushi'.
- **Vector:** Chigger.
- **Reservoir:** Rodent, birds.
- **Mode of infection:** Bite of chigger.
- **Clinical presentation:** Fever, generalised or regional lymphadenopathy, eschar at site of bite, lesion.
- **Diagnosis:** ELISA.
- On Neil Mooser or Tunica reaction there is no change seen in guinea pig on inoculation of orientia tsutsugamushi.
- **Weil Felix Reaction:** It is heterophile agglutination test. Heterophile antibodies are those that are formed due to shared or cross reactive antigen. Heterophile antigen are those which are shared over class or kingdom.

Weil Felix Reaction–Heterophile Agglutination Test Between Proteus and Rickettsial Infection

Antigens and Infections	Ox-19 of P. Vulgaris	Ox-2 of P. Vulgaris	Ox-K of P. Mirabilis
Epidemic typhus	+++	+	-
Endemic typhus	+++	+/-	-
Spotted fever (except Rickettsial fever)	++	++	-
Scrub typhus	-	-	+

- **Diagnosis:** ELISA.
- **Treatment: Drug of choice**–Doxycycline.
- Sulphonamides are Contraindicated.

58. 24 years old female is brought into emergency room with complain of fever and abdominal pain. 2 days ago she delivered a child via normal vaginal delivery at 36 weeks of gestation through her entire course of delivery she was suffering with low grade fever. On conducting detailed history it was brought to the notice by her family that patient's mother found and removed a tick from patient's neck approximately 15 days ago. Later at site of bite there developed erythema, pain

and raised mass. On examination typical lesions on her back and limbs were found (given in image below).TVS and CT scan of abdomen were conducted which showed no abnormality. On conducting blood culture in giemsa stain 'Basophillic inclusion bodies' were seen.What is the most likely pathogenic organism responsible for patient's condition?

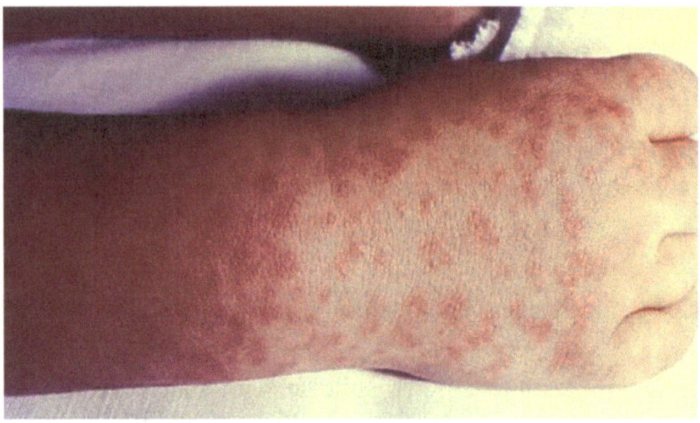

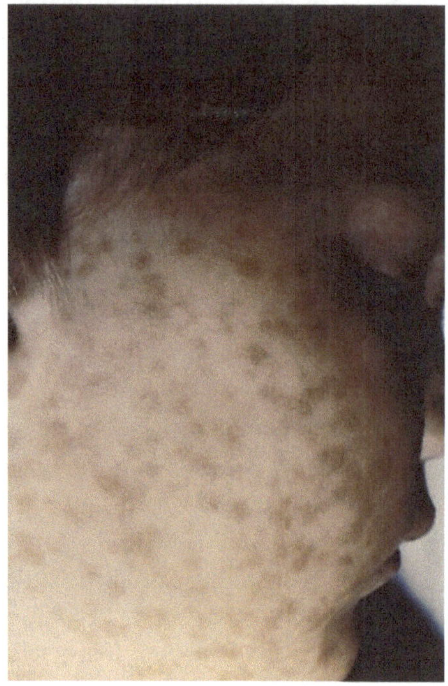

A. Coxiella burnetii
B. Orientia tsutsugamushi
C. Rickettsia prowazekii
D. Rickettsia rickettsii
E. Bartonella henselae

Answer: D. Rickettsia rickettsii

Solution

- The given case is of Rocky mountain fever which is caused by Rickettsia rickettsii.
- **Vector:** Hard tick.
- **Clinical presentation:** Characteristic rash as shown in image that start from hand and then spread to rest of body, can become hemorrhagic fever, malaise related symptoms.
- **Drug of Choice:** Doxycycline.
- In Neil Mooser or Tunica reaction Rickettsia rickettsii causes Scrotal necrosis in guinea pig upon inoculation intraperitoneally.
- For Weil Felix reaction Heterophile antigen between Proteus and Rickettsia rickettsii are Ox 19 of Proteus vulgaris and Ox2 of Proteus vulgaris.

59. 30 years old male comes with complain of consistent fever of 101°C, malaise related symptoms, myalgia and rash (as shown below in the image) for the last 4 days.

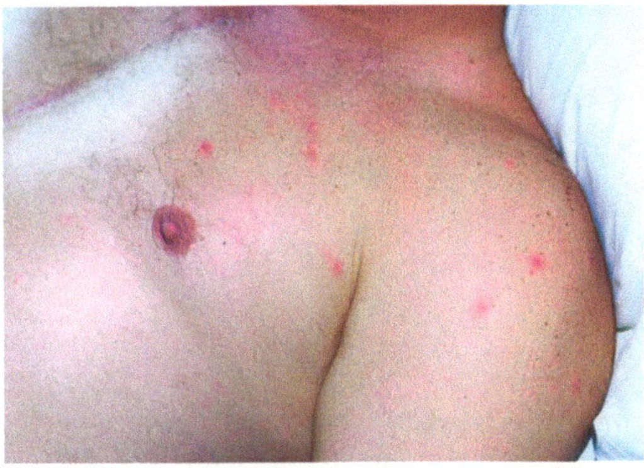

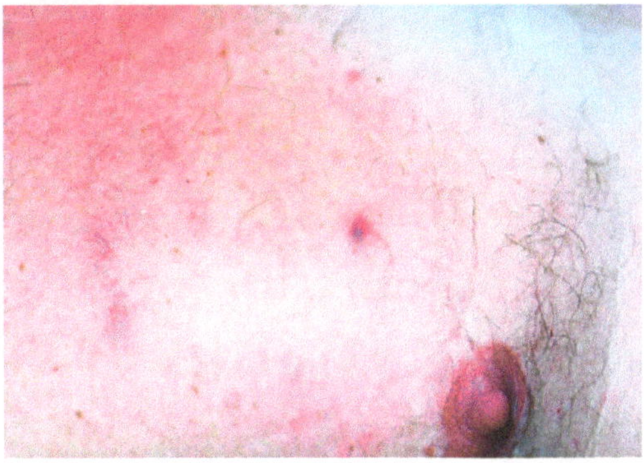

There is no associated history of nausea, vomiting, arthralgia, weight loss or diarrhea. Patient has recently visited for a jungle safari 7 days ago where he remember getting bite by a tick which even caused an eschar at site of bite as shown below:

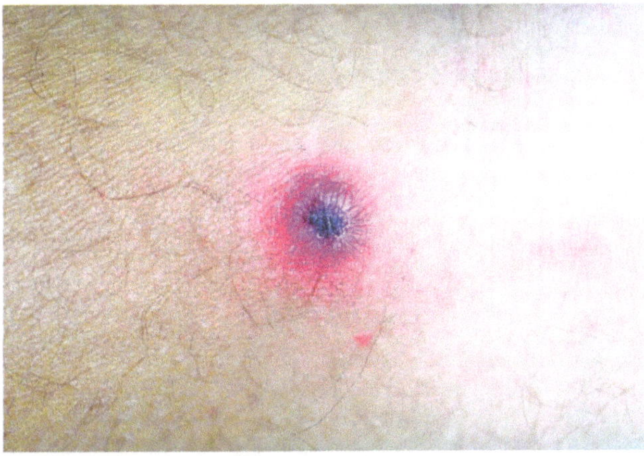

There is no other travel history. Also patient has remained on his normal diet. Patient is non alcoholic, non smoker with no known history of drug abuse. Patient has a history of hypertension for the last 6 years for which he is on ACE inhibitors since then. There is no other significant medical history or family history significant to his current presentation. On physical examination his vitals were as follows: Pulse rate of 70, Blood Pressure of 110/80, respiratory rate of 16, fever of 101.6 °C. Based on this consulting doctor conducted Complete Blood Count analysis which showed increased Neutrophils. Based on this consulting doctor send serology for Borrelia, rickettsia. Out of which IgM for Rickettsia akari came out to be positive. Which of the following is the pathogenic organism?

A. Scrub typhus

B. Rickettsia conori

C. Rickettsia akari

D. Rickettsia rickettsii

Answer: C. Rickettsia akari

60. 30 years old female present with the following presentation:

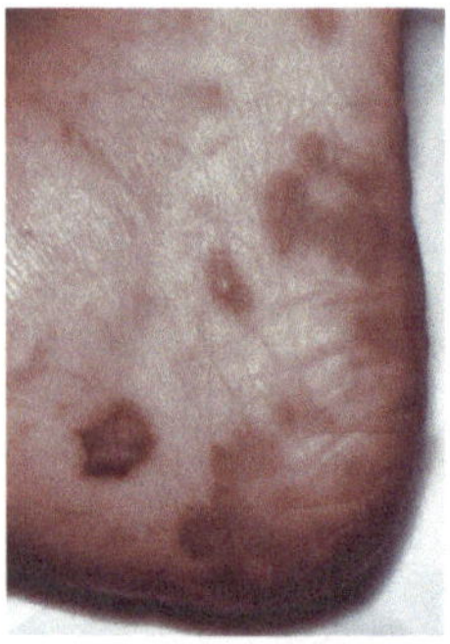

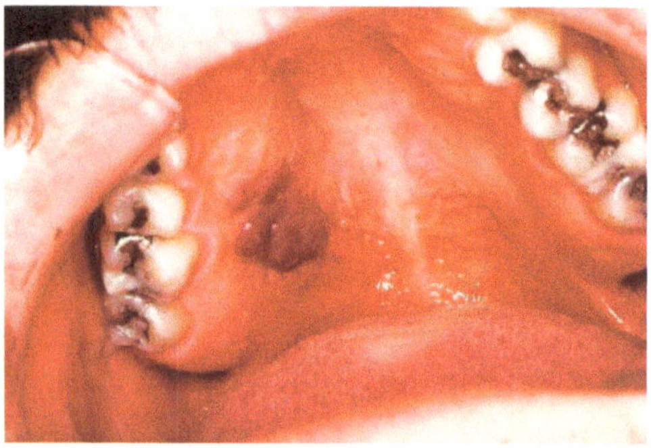

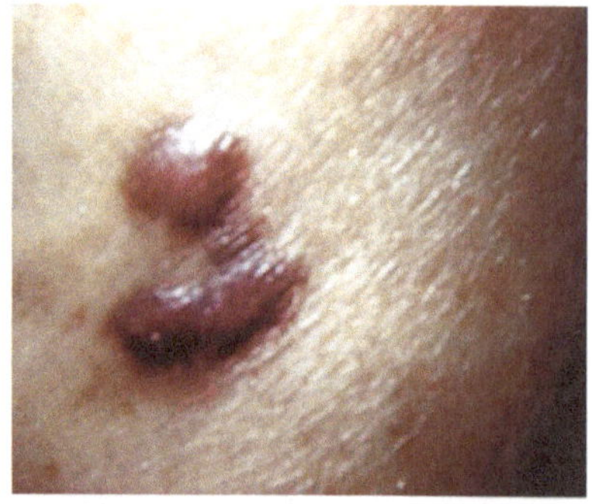

Patient is a known case of HIV and is currently on anti-retroviral regime and her most recent CD 4 counts were 106 cell/mm³. Based on this consulting doctor conducted punch biopsy for the lesion which came out to be positive for Kaposi sarcoma. Which of the following pathogenic agent would be responsible for causing Kaposi sarcoma in this patient?

A. Borrelia
B. Bordetella
C. HHV-8
D. Brucella

Answer: C. HHV-8 causes Kaposi sarcoma

61. 31 years old Gravida 3 para 3 gave birth and child was born with petechial rash as shown in image, jaundice and hepatosplenomegaly following presentation:

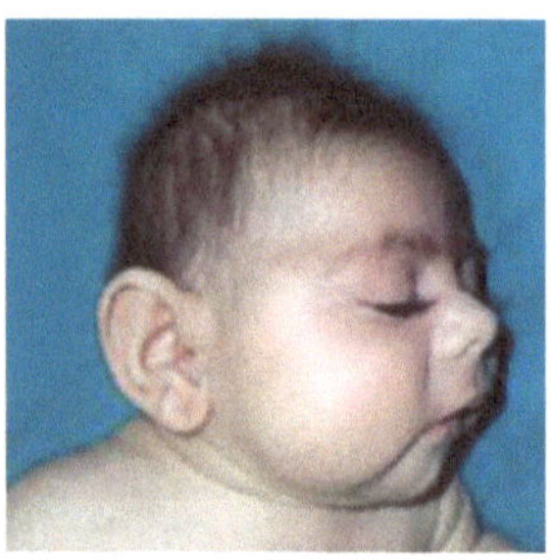

Source: Işikay S, Yilmaz K. Congenital cytomegalovirus infection and finger anomaly License:Creative Commons Attribution-ShareAlike 4.0 International license

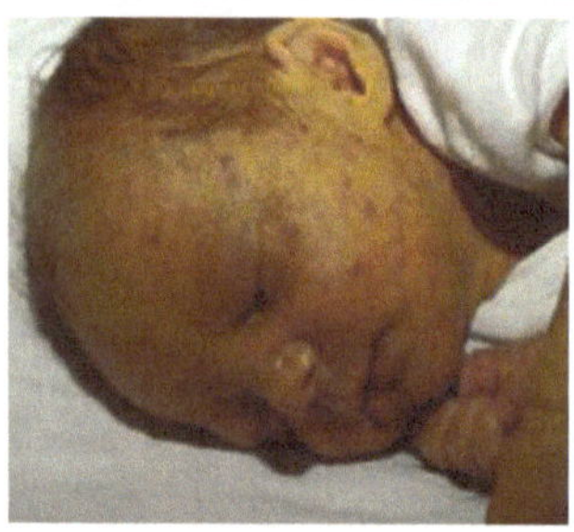

Source: CDC/Jacob Johan; License: Creative Commons Attribution-ShareAlike 4.0 International license

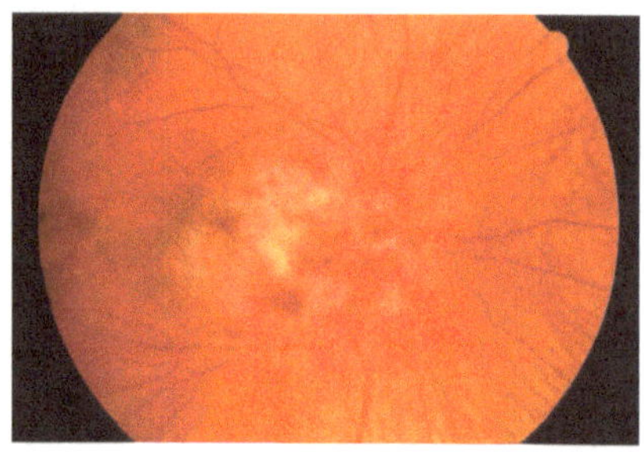

Newborn underwent screening for TORCHes infection which later came out to be positive for CMV IgM and IgG.

At this stage your professor ask you which of the following is NOT correct regarding pathogenic organism?

A. It causes infectious mononucleosus like syndrome
B. Mode of infection: Spread sexually, via blood transfusion or by prolonged contact with body fluid like urine or saliva

C. CMV becomes latent in secretory gland
D. In Complete Blood Count it causes decrease in Neutrophils and increase in lymphocytes
E. In immunocompromised patients it can cause manifestation like CMV colitis/esophagitis/pneumonia/hepatitis
F. It can cause vesicular eruption on dermatome supply ophthalmic branch of Trigeminal nerve

Answer: F. It can cause vesicular eruption on dermatome supply ophthalmic branch of Trigeminal nerve

Solution

- This is the case of Cytomegalic Inclusion Disease caused by CMV infection.
- CMV infection is part of TORCHes infection.
- Mode of transmission for CMV is prolonged contact with body fluid like urine and saliva, transfusion of blood or blood products and across placenta.
- Site of latency for CMV is salivary gland, kidney.
- It occurs when pregnant female gets infected with CMV infection and infection transmitted across placenta to fetus causing 'Cytomegalic Inclusion Disease'. It is called Cytomegalic Inclusion Disease because marked nuclear inclusion bodies in enlarged infected cells.
- **Characteristic Features of Cytomegalic Inclusion Disease:**
    1. Petechial rash.
    2. Jaundice.
    3. Hepatosplenomegaly.
    4. IUGR.
    5. Chorioretinitis.
    6. Deafness.
    7. Microcephaly.
    8. Periventricular calcification.
- Chorioretinitis caused by CMV gives characteristic 'pizza pie retinopathy' or 'Cottage cheese and sauce appearance' which is because of exudate and hemorrhage.
- **Diagnosis: Postnatal:** Serology–IgM antibody increase detected by ELISA.
- **Prenatal:** Diagnosis conduct PCR or culture on amniotic fluid.
- **Treatment** for CMV infection is intravenous ganciclovir.

62. Four college going students arrive in your hospital for blood donation. After collecting their blood your professor ask you, what are advantages of refrigerated blood after collecting? Your answer should be:

A. Treponema pallidum variety pallidum is killed at 4°C in 1-3 days hence we refrigerate blood to prevent transfusion of syphilis
B. HIV can be killed at 4°C hence we refrigerate to prevent transmission of HIV
C. Neisseria is killed at 4°C hence we refrigerate to prevent transmission of Neisseria related infections

Answer: A. Treponema pallidum variety pallidum is killed at 4°C in 1-3 days hence we refrigerate blood to prevent transfusion of syphilis

63. Forty years old male is transferred to your hospital from tertiary care center with worsening of jaundice for the last 1 month. Patient is non smoker, non alcoholic with no travel history. Patient denies commencing any recent drug intake, he did gave history of unprotected intercourse with unknown partner. Patient have normal copper level, also is negative for any hepatitis virus. On examination there were generalised lymphadenopathy (firm and non tender), also there were lesion in moist are like axilla, anogenital mucosa and oral mucosa as given below. Also there were mucous patches in oral and anogenital mucosa given below in image.

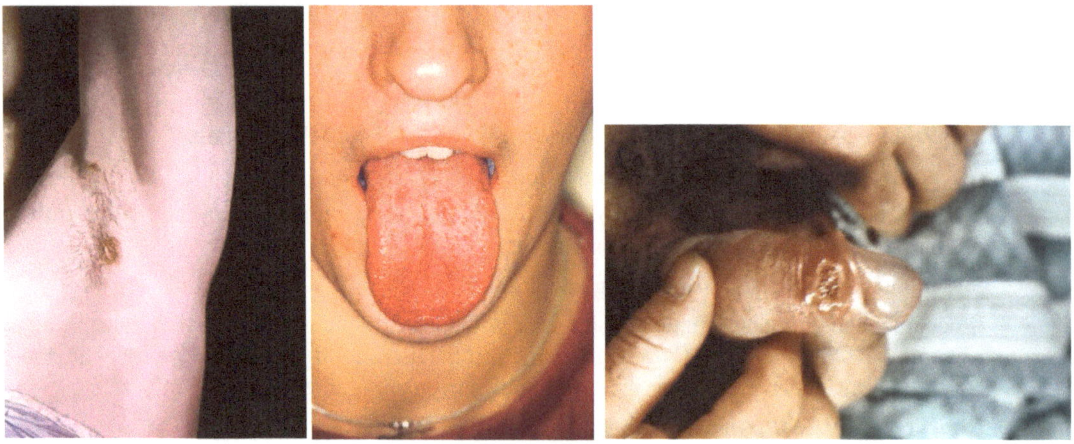

Based on given findings what type of motility is exhibited by pathogenic organism?

A. Twitching motility
B. Corkscrew motility
C. Lashing motility
D. Darting motility

Answer: B. Corkscrew motility

Solution

- The given case is that of syphilis caused by 'Treponema pallidum subsp pallidum'.
- Treponema pallidum subsp pallidum is Gram-negative spiral shaped organism.
- Treponema pallidum subsp pallidum is 'Obligate intracellular bacteria' which can't be cultivated on cell free media and hence for cultivation. It is grown on 'Rabbit testis'.
- Treponema pallidum causes syphilis which spreads only by sexual mode of transmission.
- **Incubation period:** 9-90 days.
- Treponema pallidum subsp pallidum exhibits 'Corkscrew motility'.
- As far as clinical presentation is concerned there are 4 stages of syphilis:
  1. **Primary stage:** Characterised by 'Hard/hunterian chancre'.
     - o Along with regional lymphadenopathy (firm and non tender).
     - o Symptoms resolve in 4-8 weeks.
  2. **Secondary stage:** Generally occurs 2-8 weeks after appearance of hard chancre.
     - o *Symptoms:* Generalised lymphadenopathy, Macular/papular rash that begins from trunk and proximal extremities and gradually spread all over body.

- Next manifestation of secondary stage is 'condyloma lata' generally occurs in moist areas like axilla, anogenital region, oral mucosa.
- Most infectious lesion of syphilis is 'Condyloma lata'.
- Another characteristic manifestation of Syphilis is having 'Mucous patches', mostly seen in oral and anogenital mucosa.
- Less often but in this stage patient can also suffer from:
  1. Hepatitis
  2. Nephrotic syndrome
  3. Meningitis
  4. Arthritis, periostitis
  5. Chorioretinitis, uveitis
- This stage will resolve in few months and enter in stage of latency.
- Serology positive but no manifestation.

Types of Motility of Different Organisms

Motility	*Organism*
Darting	Vibrio, Campylobacter
Corkscrew	Spirochetes
Tumbling	Listeria
Gliding	Mycoplasma
Stately	Clostridium
Swarming	Proteus
Lashing	Saprophytic spirochetes
Twitching	Trichomonas
Falling leaf	Giardia lamblia

64. 26 years old pregnant female at 5 weeks of gestation comes with a complain of vaginal lesion as shown below.

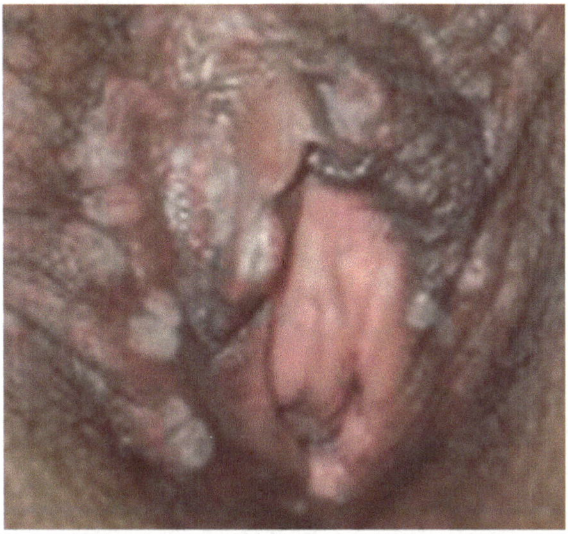

2 weeks ago she presented with complain of fever and malaise related symptoms. On examination there were inguinal region lymphadenopathy. Based on this doctor is suspicious for syphilis and sends the lesion scrapings for microscopy. Ideally which stain should be used by pathologist? (Multiple answers can be correct).

A. Negative ink staining (India ink or Nigrosin)
B. Silver impregnation (Fontana's stain or Levaditi stain)
C. Gram smear
D. ZN stain
E. Kinyoun stain
F. Rhodamine auramine stain

Answer: A and B Negative ink stain (India ink or Nigrosin); Silver impregnation (Fontana's stain or Levaditi stain)

Solution

- The given case is of syphilis caused by Treponema pallidum subsp pallidum which is obligate intra-cellular gram-negative spiral shaped organism, so can't be observed in gram smear.
- Treponema pallidum subsp pallidum exhibits 'Corkscrew motility'.
- These are spread sexually.
- **Incubation period:** 9-90 days.
- The given image in the question is that of 'Hard chancre or Huntarian chancre' occurring at 5 weeks of gestation.
- For Microscopy of these organisms we use:
  1. **Negative ink staining:** Generally used for delicate organism to study cell morphology. In negative ink staining background slide of microbial organism is stained.

     Examples: India ink or Nigrosin.
  2. Observe under dark-field microscope or phase contrast microscope.
  3. Use of prolonged giemsa stain which gives 'Rose pink spirals'.
  4. Use of silver impregnation (structure appears black in colour)–Fontana's stain (for fluid) or Levaditi stain (for tissue like biopsy).

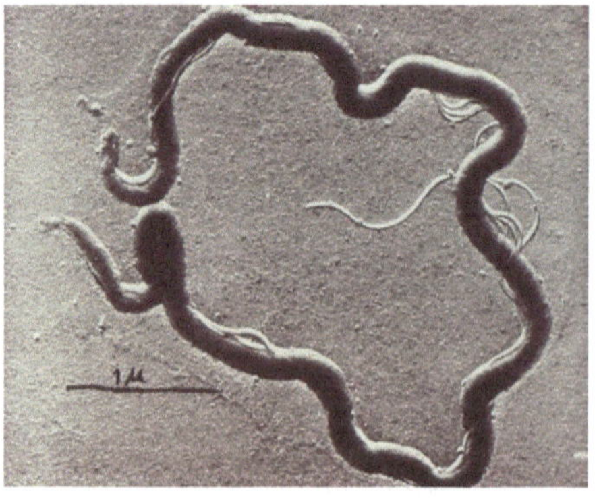

Dark-field microscopy showing spiral shaped Treponema pallidum

65. 40 years old male comes with multiple complaints of soft granulomatous tumor like growth on his neck and oral cavity for the last 10 days (shown in Figure 1), continuous decrease in vision for the last 2 days in his left eye along with Bladder incontinence and gait abnormality for the last 1 day. He has no history of trauma or previous pathology in the eye. He is diabetic for the last 12 years. He don't have history of any drug abuse but he do have a history of unprotected coital activity with commercial sex worker 2 years ago. On examination he was found to have normal memory, his pupil didn't constrict to light but did constrict to accommodation. On neurological examination patellar reflex was found to have hyperreflexia, his gait was also found to be abnormal and was having 'wide gait' abnormality. In ophthalmological examination there was dense white gaze of central region of retina along with cherry red spot at yellow spot of retina (image is given in Figure 2). Upon cardiovascular examination there was Soft, high pitched, early diastolic decrescendo murmur heard at Erb's point at end of expiration. Based on this history and examination what would be the Investigation of Choice in this patient? (Multiple answers can be correct).

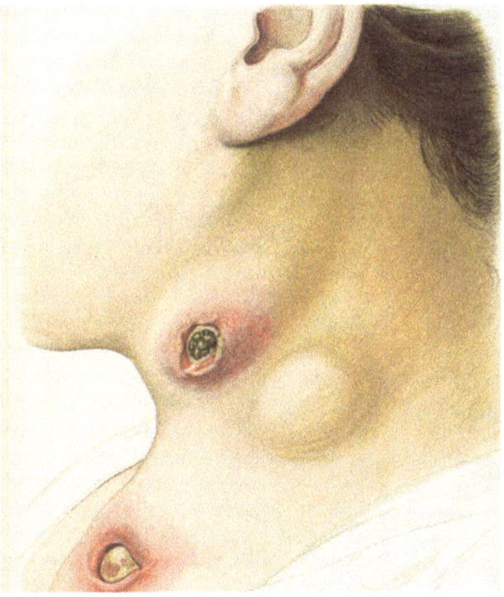

Figure 1

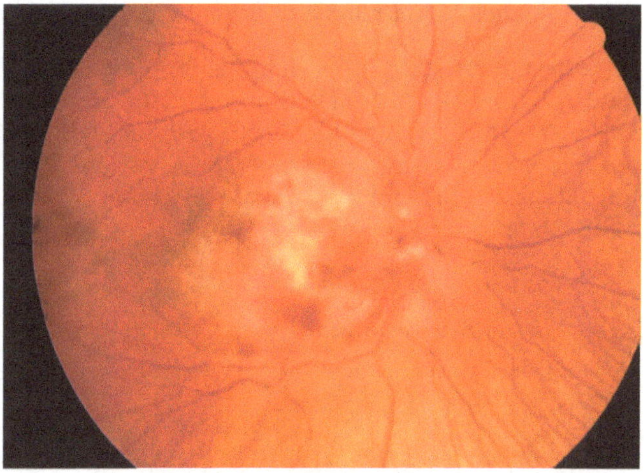

Figure 2

Source: Wikipedia; Author: Wellcome Library, London:

A. Microscopic method using Negative ink staining

B. CSF specimen's Venereal Disease Research Laboratory Test

C. CSF specimen's Indirect Fluorescent Treponema Pallidum Absorption Test

D. Microscopic visualisation using dark-field microscope or prolonged giemsa staining

Answer: B and C

Solution

- The given case is of tertiary stage of Syphilis. Syphilis is caused by obligate intracellular, gram-negative spiral shaped organism called Treponema pallidum subsp pallidum.
- Syphilis is spread sexually.

- Tertiary stage syphilis appears 5-30 years after primary manifestation of Syphilis.
- **Characteristics of tertiary stage of Syphilis are:**
  1. **Gumma:** On skin it appears as punched out ulcer.
     - o It can also appear on other sites like Bones that will lead on to fractures.
     - o Gummas can also appear on liver or other Visceral organs as well.
  2. Neurosyphilis is involvement of CNS that can be due to 'End arteritis' causing obliterating supply of blood to brain, causing symptoms like hemiparesis, hemiplegia, sensory neural hearing loss, blindness and aphasia.

     Or CNS involvement can be due to destruction of neuron, causing symptoms like Personality disorder, disorder of affect, Hyperreflexia, sensorium that cause hallucinations, delusion, Argyll Robertson pupil, disorder of intellect, speech, Tabes dorsalis (bladder incontinence, paresthesia, wide gait).
  3. There can also be Cardiovascular Syphilis due to end arteritis obliterans of vasa vasorum, aortitis, saccular aortic aneurysm, aortic regurgitation.

66. 33 years old male came to the hospital for blood donation and was found to be HIV and VDRL positive. He has a history of multiple pathological fractures. Upon taking detailed history patient tells that he had lesion on his penis 7 years ago which resolved on its own in few weeks without any intervention.There is no other significant history. On physical examination there is 'soft' high pitch decrescendo murmur heard at Erb's point. What is the Treatment of choice for this patient for Syphilis?

A. Single dose of Benzathine penicillin

B. 3 doses of Benzathine penicillin

C. First line Treatment should be Doxycycline for 2 weeks

D. First line Treatment should be Doxycycline for 4 weeks

Answer: B. 3 doses of Benzathine penicillin

Solution

- In the given patient is having signs and symptoms of tertiary stage of Syphilis like having murmur for aortic regurgitation, multiple pathological fractures are most probably due to gumma on bones.

Treatment for Syphilis:

- **Drug of choice:** Penicillin.
- **Early syphilis:** Single dose of Benzathine penicillin.
- **Late syphilis:** 3 doses of Benzathine penicillin.
- In case of penicillin allergy is Doxycycline 2 weeks for Early Syphilis and 4 weeks for Late Syphilis.
- In pregnancy Doxycycline is contraindicated therefore first line of treatment remains to be Benzathine penicillin but if patient is allergic to penicillin then 'Sensitisation of penicillin is recommended'.
- Treatment for neurosyphilis is Crystalline penicillin for 2 weeks.
- If patient is allergic to it then do sensitisation of penicillin.

Note:

- Antibiotics that are contraindicated in pregnancy are Streptomycin, Kanamycin, Tetracycline, fluoroquinolone.

67. 68 years old female is brought to ER with primary complain of progressive dyspnea, altered mental status, confusion for the last 5 days and mild chest pain on coughing for the last 2 days. 1 month back patient underwent renal transplant because of Chronic Kidney Disease caused by her uncontrolled diabetes, when patient was 9 years old she suffered with Varicella zoster infection. Patient is non smoker, non alcoholic with no known drug abuse. On monitoring vitals of patients there was increase pulse of 120, Blood pressure was 150/90, oxygen was 82% and temperature of 99.8°F. Patient is currently on metformin, glifozins and cyclosporines. On conducting physical examination it was brought to notice that patient had crop like growth of unilocular vesicular eruption in an area of 5-6 cm with surrounding erythema on lateral lower left abdomen T12 dermatome. Based on history and physical examination attending doctor conducts X-ray and sends the scrapings of base of vesicle for giemsa staining which showed pneumonia and 'multi nucleated giant cell'. At this stage your senior doctor ask you what is the pathogenic organism and what is its site of latency?

A. HHV 2 infection; site of latency is sacral ganglion

B. HHV 1 infection; dorsal root ganglion

C. HHV 1 infection; Trigeminal ganglion

D. HHV 3 infection; Trigeminal ganglion

Answer: D. HHV 3 infection; Trigeminal ganglion

Solution

- This is the case of shingles caused by zoster virus (HHV 3) reactivation due to suppressed immunity because of Transplant.
- HHV-3 or Varicella zoster virus is known to cause 'varicella infection or chickenpox' in case of primary infection and shingles/zoster in case of secondary infection.
- **Risk Factors:**
  1. Age > 60.
  2. HIV infection.
  3. Hematological malignancy.
  4. Transplant recipients.
- Site of latency of varicella zoster virus is 'Dorsal root ganglion' or 'Trigeminal ganglion'.
- **Clinical presentation:** Vesicular eruption with erythema (dew drop on rose petal) most commonly seen at T3-L2 dermatome.
- **Diagnosis:** Scrapings of base of vesicle and staining with giemsa stain or methylene blue showing Tzanck cells.
- **Serological methods:** ELISA and Fluorescent antibody to Membrane Antigen.
- **Treatment:** Valacyclovir/Acyclovir.
- To prevent reactivation of varicella zoster provide elderly (more than 50 years old) with 'Zostavax'.

68. 65 years old female comes to Emergency room with complain of jaundice, pedal edema, nausea, vomiting, weakness, shortness of breath. All these symptoms started 12 hours ago have continued to worsen. Patient was diagnosed with CML at age of 62 and was on Tyrosine kinase inhibitor Imatinib. 4 months ago she voluntarily stopped Imatinib treatment due to major depression. 10 days back she had fever, myalgia, arthralgia, along with redness in eye but she decided not to visit hospital and her condition gradually improved with home treatment. Patient have continuous exposure to fecal matter and urine of her pet dog. Doctor conducts chest X-ray and Renal Function Test that showed pneumoniae and high level of creatinine. High level of creatinine, pneumoniae, pedal edema is indicative of Acute Renal Failure. On conducting dark-field microscopy for her urine sample following organism was found.

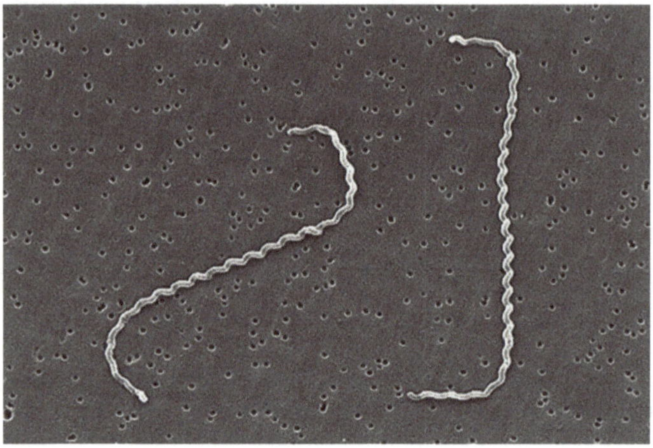

Which of the following is NOT correct regarding causative organism?

A. Most important reservoir is dog

B. It is gram-negative closely wound spiral shaped organism

C. It is 'Shepherd Crook' or umbrella handle appearance

D. It manifest 'Dinger ring' in EMJH medium

E. Disease is associated with 3 R's Rats, Rice fields and Rainfall

Answer: A. Most important reservoir is dog

Solution

- In this case patient is immunocompromised due to Imatinib Treatment. Also since patient has exposure to her dog's fecal matter making her more prone for Weil's disease or Ictero hemorrhagic fever.
- Weil's disease or Ictero hemorrhagic fever caused by leptospira which is gram-negative spiral shaped organism.
- Leptospira is 'Shepherd Crook' or umbrella shaped organism.
- Microscopically leptospira is demonstrated with dark-field microscopy, Negative staining, silver impregnation.
- Cultivation media – EMJH.
- There is formation of ring beneath surface called Dinger's ring.

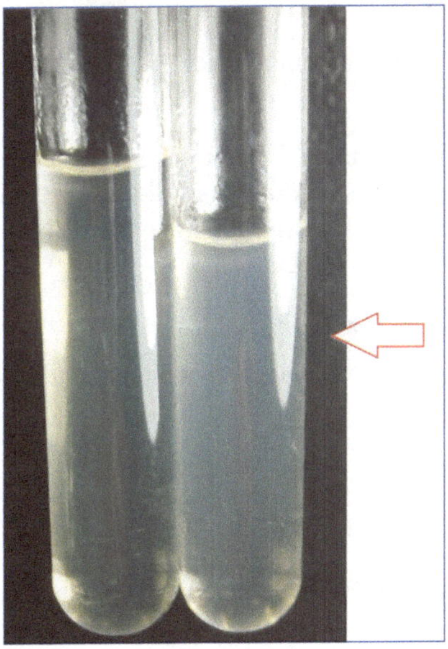

Dinger's ring

- Most important reservoir is 'Rats'.
- Other reservoir can be wild mammals and domestic animals.
- **Mode of Infection:** Percutaneous/mucous membrane exposure to urine contaminated water.
- Leptospira Infection can develop into 3 scenarios:
    1. Asymptomatic (there can be asymptomatic colonization of collecting tubules of kidney).
    2. Anicteric febrile illness.
    3. Weil's disease or Ictero hemorrhagic fever.
- Weil's disease or Ictero hemorrhagic fever has incubation period of 2-10 days.
- Weil's disease is Biphasic.
    1. Stage of bacteremia.
    2. Immunological state.
- **Stage of bacteremia:** Myalgia, fever, arthralgia, conjunctival suffusion, rashes.
- **Immunological stage (second week):** Severe headache, jaundice, Acute renal failure, encephalopathy, hemorrhages, conjunctival infection, muscle pain in calves and thighs, relative bradycardia, cutaneous and visceral hemorrhage, rhabdomyolysis in 50% patients.
- **Mortality**–15%.

Diagnosis:

- **Blood:** Positive for first week; we can do cultivation, microscopy, animal inoculation, NAAT's.
- **Urine:** Positive for second week; we can do cultivation, microscopy, animal inoculation, NAAT's.
- Serology is positive for second week.
- **Genus Specific Test:** Complement Fixation Test/Immunofluorescence Antibody Test: Patoc 1 strain for leptospira biflexa.
- **Microscopic agglutination test:** Serotype Specific antibody.

Treatment:

- **Milder cases:** Doxycycline/ampicillin/Amoxicillin moderate/severe-I/V Penicillin/Ceftriaxone/Cefotaxime/Doxycycline.

69. 27 years old male presents with complain of right hypogastric pain, jaundice, myalgia, conjunctivitis and cutaneous lesion as shown below for the last 10 days. Patient is a sewage worker. Upon further work up causative organism was found to be leptospira. Which of the following is NOT correct regarding pathogenic organism?

A. Generally infects sewage worker and rice field workers

B. Mode of Infection is percutaneous or mucus membrane exposure to urine contaminated water

C. It can cause rhabdomyolysis

D. Drug of Choice is Praziquantel

Answer: D. Drug of Choice is Praziquantel

70. 45 years old male brought to hospital with complain of headache, fever along with intermittent shivering cold spell, generalised joint pain and progressive rash. On examination there is generalised lymphadenopathy and raised lesion on back 16×18 cm in size (as given in image below). He gives a history of visiting USA on a holiday trip 10 days back where he carried out number of activities like jungle safari, mountaineering and surfing.

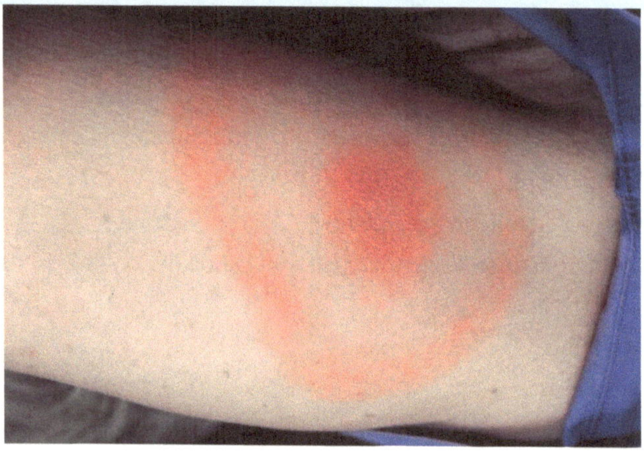

Which of the following is NOT correct regarding causative organism?

A. It is caused by gram-negative irregular spiral shaped organism called Borrelia

B. Vector–Ixodid

C. Lesion in primary stage of Lyme's disease is called Chronic Erythema Migrans or Bull's eye lesion

D. It does not affect CVS or CNS system

E. Drug of choice is Doxycycline

Answer: D. It does not affect CVS or CNS system

Solution

- This is the case of Lyme disease caused by Borrelia.
- **There are 3 main subtypes of Borrelia:**
  1. Borrelia burgdorferi (Most common in USA).
  2. Borrelia afzellii (Most common in Europe).
  3. Borrelia garinii (Most common in Asia).
- Borrelia is gram-negative irregular spiral shaped organism.

Vector-Ixodid (Hard tick)

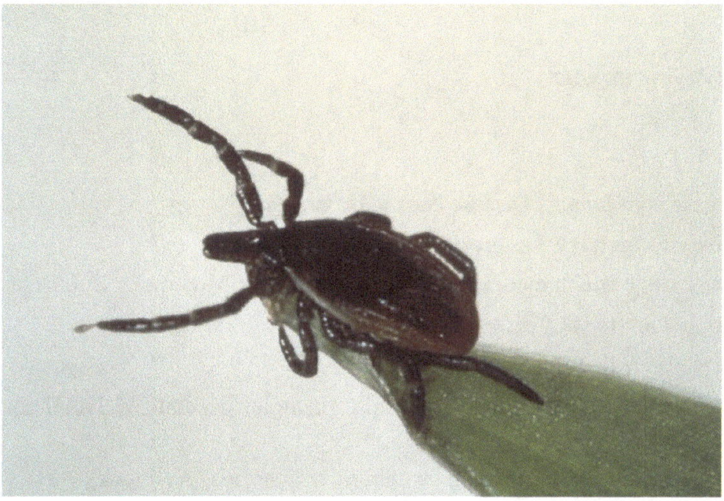

Reservoir – Rodent, Deer

- **Lyme's disease can have 3 stages:**
  1. **Primary stage:** Generally characterised by Chronic Erythema Migrans or Bull's eye rash.
  2. **Secondary stage or Stage of dissemination:** Generally characterised by General lymphadenopathy, secondary annual lesion (ECM like), migrating arthralgia, myalgia.
     - o 5-10% have meningitis or carditis (fluctuating AV block) like symptoms.
  3. Tertiary stage (Stage of persistence) appears several years later.
     - o Chronic symmetrical polyarthritis.
     - o Most common – knee.
- **Encephalopathy:** Cranial nerve palsies, cerebellar ataxia.
- **Cultivation:** BSK media.
- **Serology:** Screening–ELISA/IFAT.
  Confirmatory–Western blot.

Treatment:

- **Drug of Choice:** Doxycycline 2 weeks–2 months.
- **CVS/CNS:** I/V Ceftriaxone/Penicillin.

71. 32 years old male who is a professional marathon runner comes to primary health care physician with a complain of new onset worsening fatigue and dyspnea on exertion during his typical routine of jogging activity. He normally runs 10 miles in wood near his home 6 days a week. But recently he has noticed progressive worsening of his performance due to dyspnea, fatigue and intermittent chest tightness forcing him to have several breaks during his practice. Physician performed 12 lead EKG which showed third degree heart block. On further taking detailed history patient tells that he did had a rash in his right leg that was slightly raised target shaped erythematous patch 14 days back. Upon knowing the target shaped rash physician conducts serology for Borrelia through ELISA and confirmed by Western blot. What is the drug of choice for this case?

A. I/V Ceftriaxone
B. Doxycycline
C. Steroids
D. NSAIDs

Answer: A. I/V Ceftriaxone

Solution

- The given case is of Lyme's Disease caused by Borrelia.
- **Lyme's Disease can have 3 stages:**
    1. **Primary stage** which manifest as Erythema chronic Migrans or Bull's eye rash.
    2. **Secondary or stage of dissemination:**
        - o It is also called 'Latest great Imitator'.
        - o It manifests as migrating arthralgia, myalgia, generalised lymphadenopathy, ECM like lesion.
        - o In 5-10% patients there can be meningitis, carditis (AV block).
    3. **Tertiary stage: Stage of persistence:**
        - o It occurs several years later.
- There is chronic symmetrical polyarthritis–Most common knee.
- Encephalopathy–Cranial nerve palsy and cerebellar ataxia.

Treatment of Lyme's Disease

- **Drug of Choice**–Doxycycline for CVS and CNS associated Lyme's Disease–I/V Ceftriaxone or Penicillin.

72. 37 years old male is brought to Emergency room with complain of recurrent fever, headache, myalgia and chills for the last 8 days and jaundice for the last 2 days. Patient has returned from Jordan 5 days back from 3 weeks trip. He started having fever, headache, myalgia and other malaise related symptoms during the trip. Consulting doctor is suspicious for malaria as fever is recurrent. So he orders intern to collect the peripheral blood and send it for giemsa stained thick and thin slide. The blood was negative for parasite but there was presence of helically coiled spirochetes. So he sends serology for leptospira, Borrelia and Treponema which came out to be positive for Borrelia. What should be the Drug of Choice for this patient?

A. I/V Ceftriaxone
B. I/V Penicillin
C. Tetracycline/Macrolides
D. Quinine

Answer: C. Tetracycline/Macrolides

Solution

- The patient is suffering from Relapsing fever caused by Borrelia which is gram-negative spiral shaped organism.
- **Relapsing fever can be of 2 types:**
  1. Louse borne Relapsing fever or Epidemic Relapsing fever.
  2. Tick borne Relapsing fever or Endemic Relapsing fever.
- **Incubation period for Relapsing fever:** 2-10 days.
- **Clinical presentation:** Recurrent fever.
- In severe cases there can be: Jaundice, Hepatosplenomegaly, Lymphadenopathy, Hemorrhagic manifestation, Meningitis and hemiplegia.
- **Diagnosis:** Wet mount giemsa stain, NAAT's.
- **Culture:** BSK media.

Treatment:

- **Louse Borne Relapsing Fever:** Tetracycline/Macrolides (single dose).
- **Tick Borne Relapsing Fever:** Tetracycline/Macrolides for 10 days.
- **For CNS Involvement:** I/V Penicillin or third generation Cephalosporins.
- Relapsing fever and Lyme's disease can be very similar in presentation but both are caused by different species of borrelia.

73. 32 years old gave birth to male child at 34 weeks of gestation via normal vaginal delivery. Child was born with following presentation.

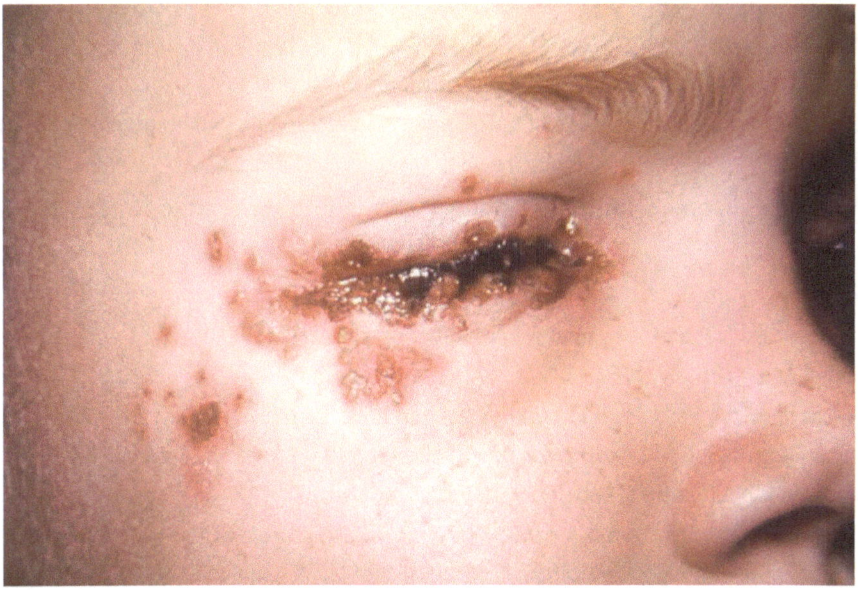

APGAR score of infant was 9. Father of the child was treated for genital lesion 7 months back as shown in the image.

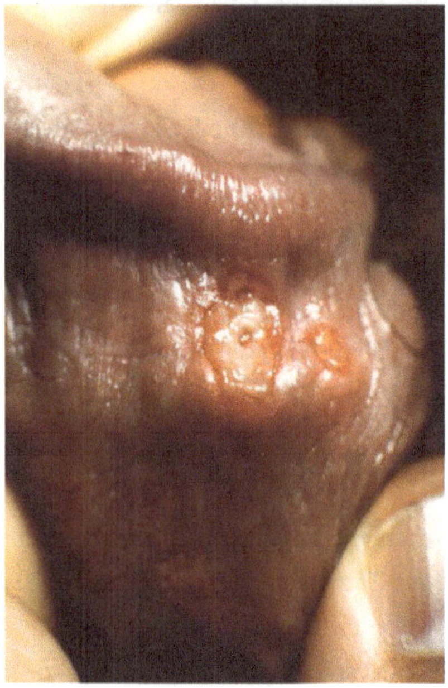

Mother was negative for rectal swab and vaginal swab for group B streptococcus. Which of the following is NOT correct regarding patient's pathology?

A. The given condition/pathology can only happen due to HSV2 infection

B. Most probably mother is the carrier of HSV-2 but asymptomatic

C. Drug of Choice is Acyclovir

D. Neonatal herpes can cause vesicular eruption on skin along with eye involvement, Encephalitis and even disseminated disease

Answer: A. The given condition/pathology can only happen due to HSV 2 infection

Solution

- The given case is that of neonatal herpes affecting skin and eye.
- Neonatal herpes is caused by HSV-2 (more common) and HSV-1.
- HSV-2 is spread by means of sexual contact and undergo latency in Sacral ganglion.
- Clinical presentation of primary and reactivation of HSV-2 remains same, i.e., genital ulcer.
- **Diagnosis:** NAAT, antigen specific immunofluorescence.
- Other diagnostic modality also include staining the scrapings of base of vesicular ulcer showing Tzank smear and eosinophilic intranuclear inclusion body.
- **Treatment:** Acyclovir.
- **Neonatal herpes can occur:**
  1. Intrapartum.

2. Perinatal transmission (most common).
3. Postnatally.

- **Clinical presentation of neonatal herpes:**
  1. Crops of vesicle eruption (shown in image).
  2. Ophthalmic involvement.
  3. Encephalitis (focal or generalised seizure, respiratory problems, abnormal tone of body, decrease reflexes).
  4. Disseminated disease.
- **Treatment:** IV Acyclovir for 6-12 months.

74. Gravida 2 para 1 female presents at 30 weeks of gestation with complain of fever and malaise related symptoms along with complain of myalgia and abdominal pain for the last 14 hours. Fever was 101°C and abdominal pain was at continuous and cramping in hypogastric region. Patient tells that she had contact with sick patient and all her family members are suffering from flu like symptoms. At this stage consulting doctor conducted Biophysical score which came out to be 7/10. Complete Blood Count analysis indicated toward bacterial infections and patient was started on ampicillin and clindamycin. As patient's fever started decreasing she was discharged from the hospital. 2 days later she returned with fever, abdominal pain and vaginal bleeding. Biophysical score was 5/10 at this stage consulting doctor decided to conduct delivery. Child was born with APGAR score of 7/10 and 8/10 at 1 minute after birth and 5 minutes after birth respectively. Post operatively mother health was stable. But 3 weeks later neonate suffered from respiratory distress, sepsis and meningitis and was put on respiratory support. Blood investigation and serology revealed presence of Listeria monocytogenes. Which of the following is NOT correct regarding the pathogenic organism?

A. It can be grown on 'Mueller Hinton agar' with sheep's blood

B. If pregnant female gets infected in first semester then it can cause abortion and still birth

C. It infects immunocompromised and immunocompetent patients equally

D. Asymptomatic colonisation in vagina causes infertility

Answer: C. It infects immunocompromised and immunocompetent patients equally

Solution

- This is the case of Listeria monocytogenes infection which is gram-positive coccal bacteria which is a facultative anaerobe.
- **General biochemical properties:**
  1. Catalase positive
  2. Oxidase negative
  3. Methyl red positive
  4. Voges-Proskauer positive

Clinical Presentation:

- It mainly affects pregnant female, infants and immunocompromised patients.
- **Common symptoms are:**
  1. Fever and malaise related symptoms.
  2. Nausea, vomiting.

3. Severe headache.
4. Diarrhea, Constipation.
5. Abdominal pain.
6. Meningitis.
7. Can even cause abortion and still birth particularly if female is infected in first trimester.
8. Neonatal infant can have abscess, pharyngitis, conjunctivitis, urethritis, meningitis and septicaemia.

Diagnosis:

1. **Culture:** Listeria monocytogenes can be grown on 'Mueller Hinton agar' with sheep's blood and forms beta hemolytic colonies.
2. Serological methods like ELISA.
3. Molecular methods PCR and NAAT's.

Treatment:

- Drugs that can be used are Ampicillin, erythromycin, Trimethoprim–Sulphmethoxazole.
- In pregnancy drugs like penicillin ampicillin and Amoxicillin are safe to use and are preferred.
- **Drug of Choice for Listeria** monocytogenes infection.

75. 10 years old male is brought by his parents with complain of mild persistent fever and severe persistent cough along with weight loss for the last 18 days. Fever has remained around 100°C, cough was dry and there have been spells of cough that has remained for more than 1 minute. Also patient has lost 3 kg in last 18 days. There is no associated history of lesions or chills or myalgia or rhinorrhea or nausea or vomiting. Child birth was uneventful via normal vaginal delivery at 37 weeks of gestation and his vaccine status is incomplete. On physical examination patient vitals were as follows pulse 82, blood pressure 123/78, respiratory rate of 20 and fever was 100.2°C. Oral examination was unremarkable with no swelling of tonsils or exudation present.

Chest examination was unremarkable with no crackle or wheezing sound there was no sign of consolidation. On conducting Complete Blood Count analysis lymphocytes were 45% along with 30% neutrophils.

Based on this consulting doctor conducted serology for Rhinovirus, influenza virus, adenovirus and Bordetella out of which Bordetella came out to be positive. At this stage your professor ask you which of the following is NOT correct regarding the pathogenic organism?

A. Preferred medium of growth is Bordet gengou glycerine potato blood agar
B. Colonies are dome shaped smooth, opaque, white in colour resembling bisected pearl or mercury drop surrounded by hazy zone of hemolysis
C. It produces pertussis that is Dermo necrotic in nature
D. It produces hemagglutinin that help in adherence to respiratory epithelium and RBC's
E. Drug of choice is Penicillin

Answer: E. Drug of choice Penicillin

Solution

- This is the case of whooping cough in an unvaccinated child.
- Whooping cough is caused Bordetella pertussis.

- Bordetella pertussis is gram-negative coccobacilli organism.
- **General biochemical characteristics:**
  1. Catalase positive
  2. Oxidase positive
  3. Urease positive
  4. Reduce nitrates
  5. Indole test positive
- It produces pertussis toxins that is highly toxic and dermo necrotic in nature.
- This toxin is responsible for generating immune response which causes lymphocytosis.
- Pertussis or whooping cough caused by Bordetella pertussis has 3 stages:
  1. **Stage 1 or catarrhal stage:** Cause running nose fever cough.
  2. **Stage 2 or paroxysmal stage:** Rapid cough with whoop at the end.
  3. **Stage 3 or convalescent stage:** Severity of cough decreases.
- Pertussis produces hemagglutinin which helps in adherence to respiratory epithelium or RBC's.
- Because of the non specific symptoms sometimes Bordetella pertussis is misdiagnosed as Mycoplasma infection (specially due to weight loss that can occur) and adenovirus infection (due to lymphocytosis).
- **Diagnosis:**
  1. Microscopy.
  2. **Culture:** Cultivation media–Border gengou glycerine potato blood agar.
     - o The colonies formed are glittering, dome shaped opaque along with surrounding hazy hemolysis.
     - o Having an appearance bisected pearl or mercury drop.
     - o Confluent growth present as 'Aluminium paint like appearance'.
  3. Cough plate method is one of the bed side method used for diagnosing pertussis done by placing plate 10-15 cm in front of mouth and patient is asked to cough.
     - o Infected droplets get impinged on the media.
  4. Serological methods like ELISA, IgA is detected by ELISA from nasopharyngeal secretions.
  5. Molecular methods like PCR or NAAT's.

Treatment:

- **Drug of Choice**–Macrolide antibiotics.
- **Vaccination**–DPT vaccine.

76. Three years old male child is brought by his parents with multiple complain of fever along with malaise related symptoms, 2 jet like vomiting, headache and neck stiffness and photophobia for the last 2 days. Fever was 101.5°C, headache was persistent and affected whole head. Patient's family belong from low socioeconomic background. Child birth was uneventful but his vaccine status is incomplete. Based on this consulting doctor conducted. His Complete Blood Count analysis and lumbar puncture which showed increased level of lymphocytes. His lumbar puncture pressure was normal and clear in appearance lymphocyte predominance, normal glucose, raised protein (but < 200 mg/dL).
Gram staining showed pink colour gram-negative rod shaped bacteria. At this stage consulting doctor send serology for Haemophilus influenzae type B which came out to be positive. Which of the following is NOT correct regarding pathogenic organism?

A. They exhibit property called Satellitism
B. Haemophilus is also known to cause chancroids
C. Type 1 Haemophilus influenzae is sub divided on the basis of hemagglutinin and neuraminidase
D. Haemophilus is known to cause purulent conjunctivitis

Answer: C. Type 1 Haemophilus influenzae is sub divided on the basis of hemagglutinin and neuraminidase

Solution

- This is the case of Haemophilus influenzae type B causing meningitis.
- Haemophilus is gram-negative rod shaped bacteria found as normal flora of respiratory tract and oral cavity.

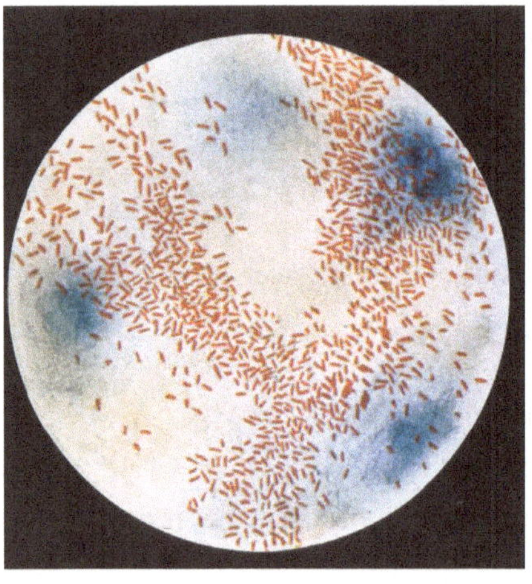

Gram stain for Haemophilus influenzae

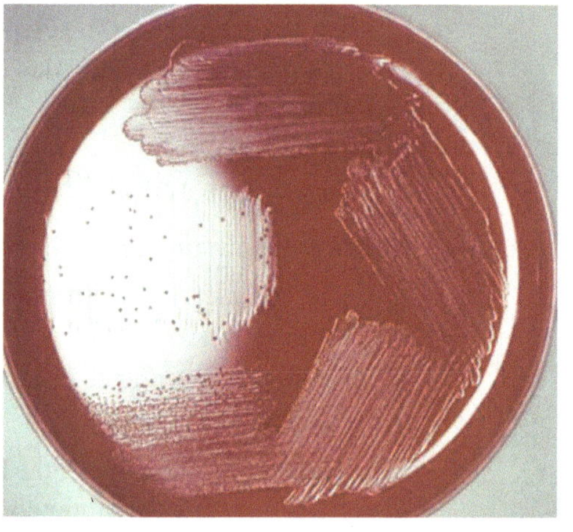

Blood agar for Haemophilus influenzae

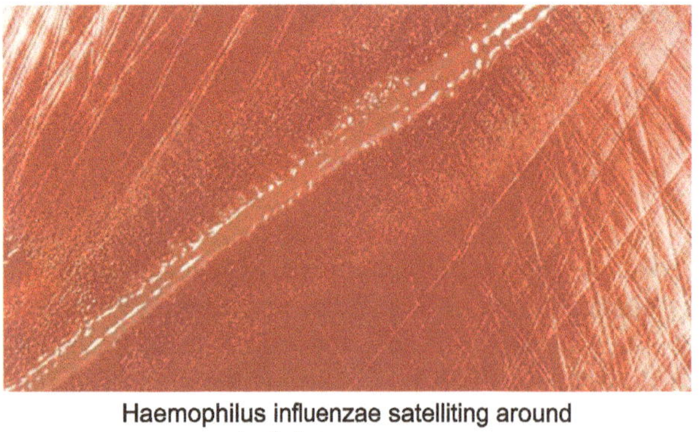

Haemophilus influenzae satelliting around staphylococcus aureus

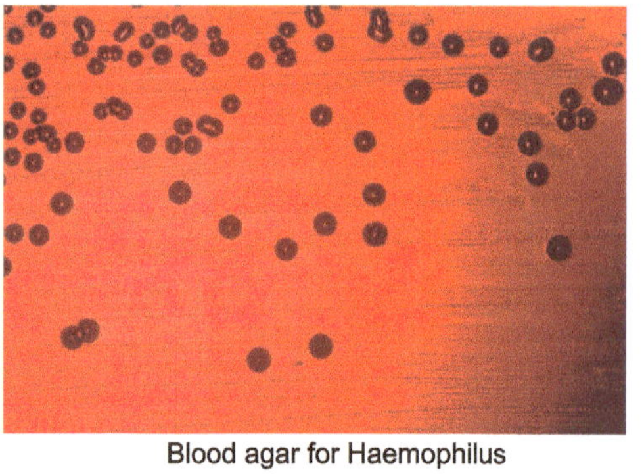

Blood agar for Haemophilus influenzae

- Some of the clinically significant Haemophilus species are:
    1. Haemophilus influenzae–Causing meningitis, epiglottitis, pneumonia etc.
    2. Haemophilus ducreyi is sexually transmitted organism causing chancroid.
    3. Haemophilus parainfluenza causes pneumonia and endocarditis.
    4. Haemophilus aegyptius causes purulent conjunctivitis or pink eye.
- **Mode of Transmission:** Via direct or indirect contact with respiratory droplets.
- **Biochemical Properties:** Catalase positive and Oxidase positive.
- Nitrate reduction test positive.
- Indole variable.
- As for staining we use 'Loffler's methylene blue'.
- As for the culture it grows on blood agar and form opaque colonies, factor 10 and factor 5 are essential for the growth.
- Haemophilus influenzae exhibit property of Satellitism that is when staphylococcus aureus is streaked across the palate containing Haemophilus influenzae larger colonies develop around streak and smaller further away.
- **Clinical Presentation:**
    1. Meningitis.
    2. Epiglottitis.
    3. Pneumonia.
    4. Arthritis.
    5. Cellulitis.
- Most of them are opportunistic infections and unvaccinated individual (specially children) are at high risk.
- **Diagnosis:**
    1. Microscopy.
    2. Serology like ELISA.
    3. Molecular methods like PCR and NAAT's.
- **Treatment:**
    - o Drugs that can be used are ceftriaxone, azithromycin, Doxycycline.

77. 52 years old male came to OPD with multiple complains of intermittent fever and malaise related symptoms for the last 2 months, back pain and weight loss for the last 1 month. Fever particularly rises nocturnally and remains under 101°C. He has lost 5 kgs in the last 1 month. There is no history of diarrhea or abnormal bowel movements. Patient is a farmer by occupation and owns cattle sells its dairy products for living. Patient is non smoker, non alcoholic with no history of drug abuse. He has remained on his usual dietary pattern. He denies being in contact with any ill patient. There is no autoimmune related family history. Patient has hypertension for the last 22 years and have been on ACE inhibitor since then. He is also having diabetes mellitus type 2 for the last 10 years and have been on metformin and glifozins since then. 7 years ago patient underwent heart valve replacement surgery. On physical examination patient face was dull, ill looking and following lesions were noticed along with nail bed hemorrhage.

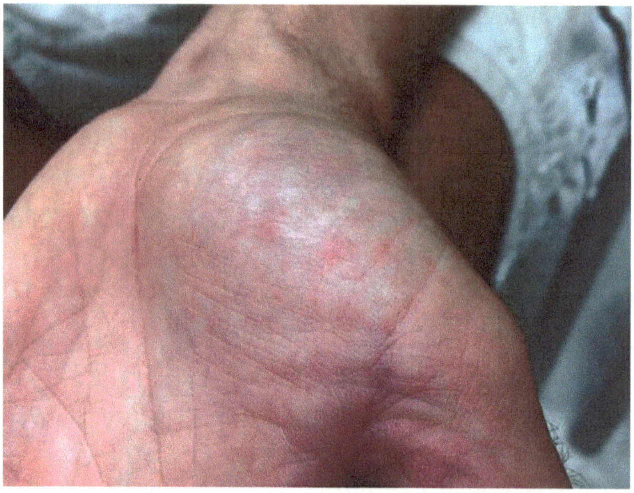

Source: Wikipedia; Author: Warfieldian

A. It is intracellular gram-negative aerobic coccobacilli

B. IMViC all tests are negative

C. Catalase and Oxidase positive

D. Urease and nitrate reduction test both are positive

E. Dinger's ring test was positive

Answer: E. Dinger's ring test was positive

Solution

- This is the case of brucella infection.
- Brucella is intracellular gram-negative coccobacilli.
- They are strict aerobe.
- **Mode of Infection:** Brucella can be transmitted via multiple ways.
    1. *Oral entry:* Particularly by consumption of contaminated raw milk product.
    2. Aerosol.
    3. Percutaneous exposure.
- **Milk Ring Test:** This is frequently used serological test to check for presence of antibodies in milk of animals.
- This is performed by adding drop of blue colour brucella antigen in test tube of whole milk and then left in water bath at 70°C for 40-50 minutes.
- If positive then antibodies present in milk and antigen agglutinate and raised with cream to form blue colour ring at top leaving milk unstained.
- If test is negative then whole milk remain stained blue.
- General biochemical test of Brucella.
- Catalase positive.

- Oxidase positive.
- Nitrate reduction test positive.
- Urease test positive.
- IMViC test all negative.

Clinical Presentation:

- **For acute brucellosis:** Muscular and articular pain, weight loss, nocturnal sweating, fever along with chills, anorexia and constipation.
- **For chronic brucellosis:** Sweating, joint pain and mild fever.
- Other manifestations that can occur are:
    1. Endocarditis.
    2. Meningitis or encephalitis.
    3. Diarrhea or constipation.
    4. Hepatosplenomegaly.
    5. Epididymo-orchitis.

Diagnosis:

- Since it is intracellular organism so microscopy is not very helpful.
    1. Serological methods like ELISA.
    2. Molecular methods like PCR.
    3. **Blood culture:** Castaneda's method.

Treatment:

- Doxycycline + Rifampin.
- Vaccine available is intradermal recommended if someone visits endemic areas.

78. Patient was brought to OPD by her parents with following presentation.

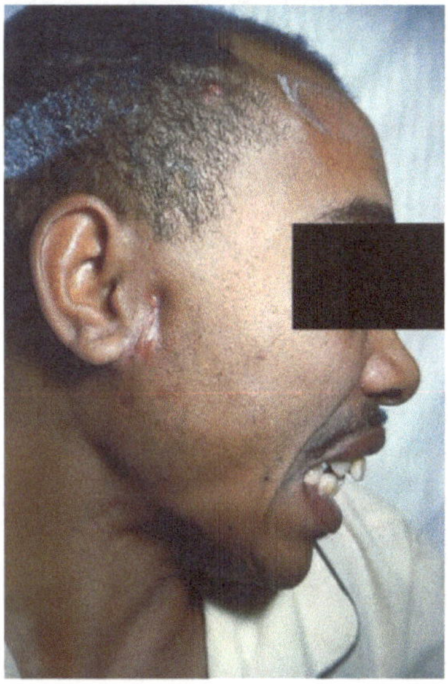

This swelling has existed for the last 20 days and there have been history of multiple pus discharge. Patient gives a history of trauma causing laceration on face 1 month back. Patient's birth history is unremarkable via normal vaginal delivery and his vaccine status is complete. Doctor decided to send aspiration cytology for examination that showed outer zone granulation and central necrosis containing multiple basophilic granules that represent lobulated micro colonies of actinomyces. What is Drug of Choice for this patient?

A. Oral penicillin for 3-6 weeks and surgical drainage

B. Azoles for 2-3 weeks and surgical

C. Praziquantel for 3 weeks and surgical drainage

D. Cotrimoxazole + linezolids

Answer: A. Oral penicillin for 3-6 weeks and surgical drainage

Solution

- This is the case of faciocervical actinomycosis.
- Actinomyces are gram-positive rod shaped, filamentous and facultative anaerobe.
- Actinomyces manifest certain fungal characteristics like producing mycelium and fry spores.
- Actinomyces constitute part of normal flora of oral cavity hence trauma in faciocervical region can cause faciocervical actinomyces.
- Hallmark feature of faciocervival actinomyces is tendency to spread regardless of anatomical barrier.

Clinical Presentation:

- Actinomyces manifest clinical presentation based upon their site of infection.
- Faciocervical actinomycosis > abdominopelvic actinomycosis > pulmonary actinomycosis.
- Pelvic actinomycosis generally occur post trauma, surgery or insertion of contraceptive device.
- As for the abdominal actinomycosis appendicitis patient particularly with perforation are at high risk of developing abdominal actinomycosis.
- Actinomycosis infection is particularly associated with the breakdown of mucous membrane.
- **As for the clinical features of abdominopelvic actinomycosis are:**
  1. Fever.
  2. Weight loss.
  3. Change of bowel habits.
  4. Sensation of mass, it presents as firm hard mass that is fixed to underlying tissue and often mistaken for tumor.
- One of the differentiating factor for abdominal mass is that tumors are generally associated with lymphadenopathy while abdominal actinomycosis generally don't present with lymphadenopathy.
- CT scan for abdominal actinomycosis generally manifest mass like lesion with focal area of decreased attenuation or thick walled cystic mass.
- Pulmonary actinomycosis occurs probably because of aspiration of oropharyngeal or gastrointestinal secretions.
- Hence often seen in alcoholics.

- **Risk factors for pulmonary actinomycosis are:**
  1. Heavy smoker.
  2. Chronic alcoholic.
  3. Conditions causing chronic cough.
  4. Poor dental hygiene.
- **Clinical features of pulmonary actinomycosis are:**
  1. Low grade fever.
  2. Cough with purulent.
  3. Blood streak sputum.
  4. Pleuritic chest pain.
- X-ray findings of pulmonary actinomycosis are unilateral peripheral patchy consolidation mainly affecting lower lobe.
- CT scan is associated with localised patchy consolidation with central area of low attenuation and associated rim enhancement, typically along with pleural membrane enhancement.

Treatment:

- **Drug of Choice:** High dose penicillin.
- Actinomyces is also sensitive to beta-lactams.

79. 42 years old male presented with complain of fever and dyspnea for the last 2 days. His fever remained 101°C persistently. He has no associated symptoms like cough, nausea or vomiting. Patient is smoker, smokes 2 packets/day for the last 20 years, non alcoholic, with no known history of drug abuse. Patient has no associated travel history in the recent past. He strongly denies of being in contact with any other ill patient. Patient is diabetic for the last 14 years and have been on metformin for the last 14 years. Patient also has a medical history for COPD for the last 6 years and have been advised salbutamol inhaler.

On physical examination patient was restless with dull looking face and bluish tinge on skin of upper limb distal phalanges (sign of cyanosis). As for his vitals his pulse rate was 92, blood pressure 152/90, respiratory rate was 23, oxygen saturation was 87% along with 102°C fever. Based on this doctor conducts chest X-ray and complete blood count analysis which showed multiple patchy consolidation in right lung, his complete blood count analysis showed neutrophils 70%, lymphocytes 20%.

Consulting doctor started patient on ampicillin along with third generation cephalosporins and conducted serology for Streptococcus, neisseria, Chlamydia, mycoplasma and legionella. All the serology came out to be negative and patient's condition deteriorated despite of antibiotics. Next morning patient started complaining of chest pain and suddenly developed 'Generalised tonic clonic seizure' in post ictal phase he had urinary incontinence. At this stage patient was referred for Brain MRI which showed presence of brain abscess in Parietal region and for chest CT chest was conducted showing presence of massive pleural edema.

This made consulting doctor highly suspecious for Nocardia and send for serology which came out to be positive. What would be the Drug of Choice for this patient?

A. Ceftriaxone
B. Cotrimoxazole + linezolid + cephalosporins
C. Ciprofloxacin
D. Praziquantel

Answer: B. Cotrimoxazole + linezolid + cephalosporins

Solution

- Nocardia is thin aerobic gram-positive bacilli that form branching filament.
- The bacteria is stained irregularly and appears beaded on gram smear.
- Nocardia is considered to be positive acid fast on ZN stain due to presence of mycolic acid in cell wall.
- Nocardia gives beaded appearance on acid fast staining.
- Nocardia is known to cause disease in both immunocompromised and immunocompetent.
- **3 common causing human Nocardia species are:**
  - o N. asteroides.
  - o N. brasiliensis (mainly cause cutaneous infection cellulitis and abscess).
  - o N. farcinica (mainly cause cutaneous infection cellulitis and abscess).
  - o N. caviae.
  - o N. abscessus (known to cause pulmonary and brain infection).
  - o **Mode of Transmission:** Inhalation of air borne bacilli or traumatic inoculation into the skin.

Clinical Presentation:

1. Multiple patchy consolidation in lungs.
2. Necrotising pneumonia can also cause cavitation.
3. Brain ulcer.
4. Cutaneous lesion.
5. Secondary Parkinsonism.

Diagnosis:

1. **Microscopy methods:** By staining infected specimen.
   - o Mainly specimen used are sputum, pleural fluid and on rare occasions even pulmonary biopsy.
2. **Culture media:** Sabouraud's glucose agar, blood agar forms smooth, moist colonies with powdery surface.
3. **Molecular methods** like NAAT's.
4. **Serological methods:** ELISA.

Treatment:

- Patient may be required to take multiple antibiotics and even for months.
- **Drug of Choice:** Cotrimoxazole + linezolids + cephalosporins.

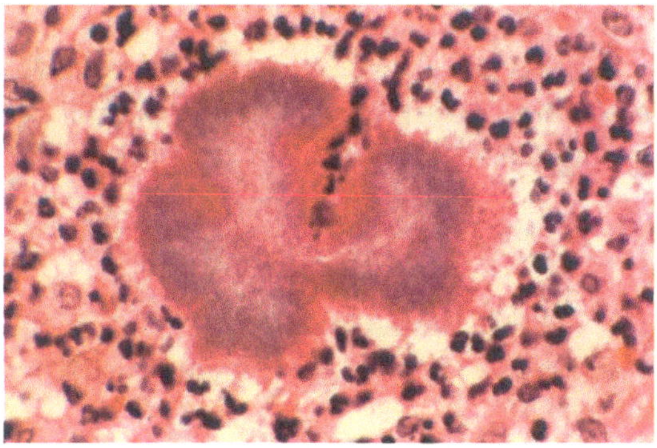

Nocardia in H and E stain

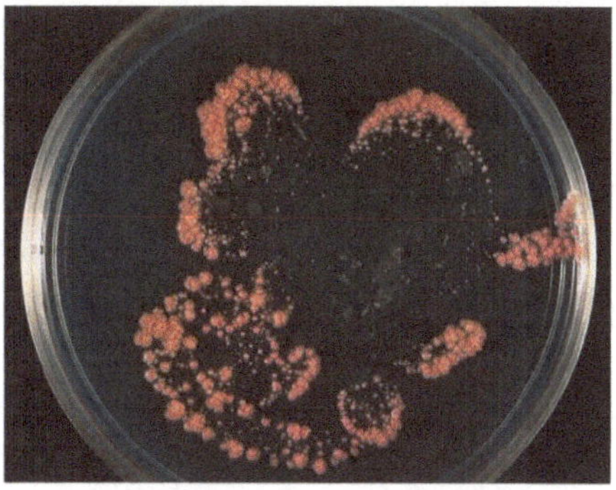

Nocardia in growth medium

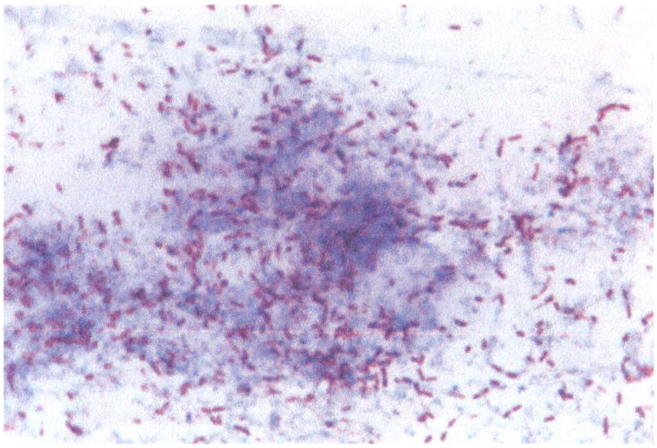

Nocardia in acid fast stain

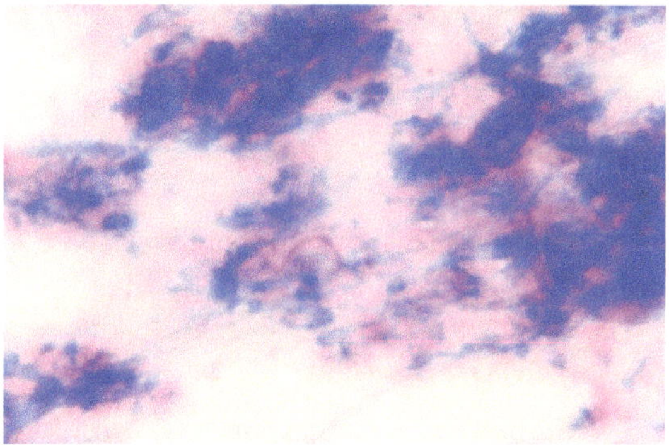

Nocardia in acid fast stain in pus medium

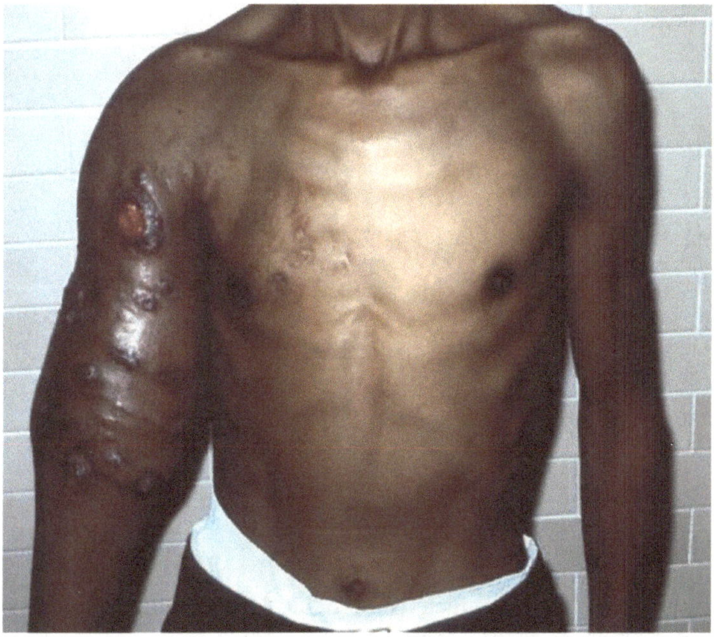

Nocardia causing cellulitis inflammation

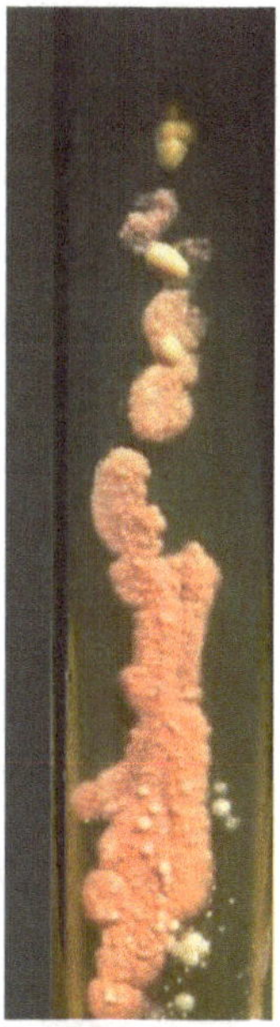

SDA showing Nocardia growth

80. 29 years old male is brought to Emergency room unconscious. His family says that he has been suffering from severe diarrhea for the last 20 days. Diarrhea was non bloody, with no mucous. On physical examination his pulse rate was 60, blood pressure was 105/68 respiratory rate is 14. Patient was started on 5% dextrose solution. Patient family tells that he has no associated travel history and have mainly stuck to daily routine diet. Patient is non alcoholic, non smoker with no known history of drug abuse. On conducting his Complete Blood Count analysis his Eosinophils was elevated and decreased CD-4 counts.

Based on this doctor conducts serology for HIV, strongyloid stercoralis, ascaris, hookworm, Cryptosporidium out of which HIV and Cryptosporidium came out to be positive. Based on this what would be Treatment of Choice for this patient?

A. Cotrimoxazole
B. Albendazole
C. Metronidazole
D. Nitazoxanide

Answer: D. Nitazoxanide

Solution

- This is the case of cryptosporidium which is generally found in HIV patients.
- Cryptosporidium is known to cause persistent diarrhea in HIV patients.

General Characteristics:

- **Habitat:** Small intestine mucosal cells.
- **Mode of infection:** Feco-oral route.
- Cryptosporidium cyst survive regular chlorination of water.

Clinical Presentation:

1. Abdominal pain.
2. Nausea and vomiting.
3. In immunocompetent it cause self resolving diarrhea.
4. In immunocompromised it causes persistent diarrhea.

Diagnosis:

1. Stool specimen is stained by kinyoun or modified ZN stain which shows presence of sporulated oocyte.
2. Immunofluorescence.
3. NAAT's.

Drug of Choice:

- Nitazoxanide.
- Cyclospora and cystoisospora most of general characteristics, clinical presentation and diagnosis remains same except for their treatment. Drug of Choice is Cotrimoxazole.

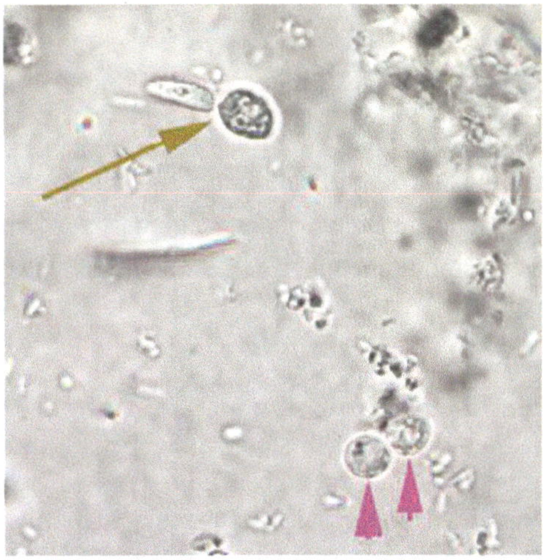

Cryptosporidium oocyte in wet mount

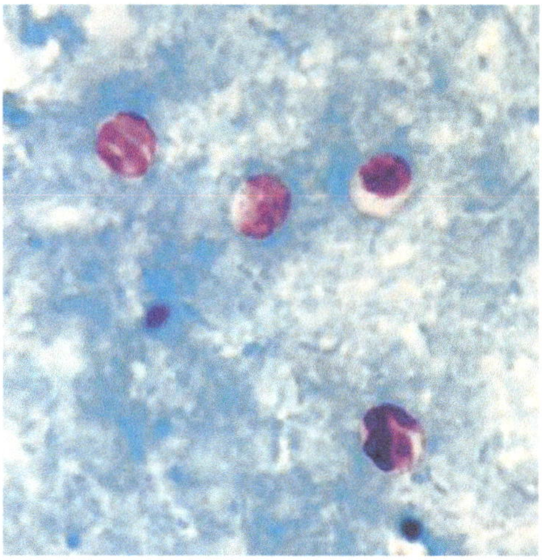

Cryptosporidium oocyte stained with modified acid fast

81. 37 years old male comes with complain of progressively increasing generalised edema particularly in periorbital region, wrist and ankles along with loss of appetite and weight gain. Patient is HIV infected individual and is on antiviral drug for the last 14 months and has been infected by plasmodium malariae causing malaria 4 times in last 1 year. On taking detailed history patient told that he has been noticing foamy froth formation after urinating. On conducting urine analysis dip stick test showed the presence of albumin in urine. Consulting doctor was suspicious of quartan malarial nephropathy. Which of the following is NOT correct regarding diagnosis of malaria?

A. Microscopy is gold standard for diagnosing Plasmodium malariae

B. Micro-hematocrit tube is more sensitive than Microscopy

C. Rapid diagnostic test detect antigen in patient's blood

D. Thin blood film/smear is used for detecting presence of parasite and rough estimate of parasitemia while thick blood film/smear is used for species identification and exact quantification of parasitemia

Answer: D. Thin blood film/smear is used for detecting presence of parasite and rough estimate of parasitemia while thick blood film/smear is used for species identification and exact quantification of parasitemia

Solution

- The given case is of Quartan malarial nephropathy which generally occurs due to chronic or repetitive infection by Plasmodium malariae.
- In this case there is formation of immune complexes which gets deposited in glomeruli leading to Nephrotic Syndrome.

Diagnosis:

- **Microscopy:** It is a gold standard for diagnosis.
- **Sensitivity:** 5 parasites/microlitre.
- **Thick blood film/smear:** It is prepared by air drying for 30 minutes.
- Its sensitivity is 5 parasites/microlitre.

- Used for detecting presence of parasite.
- It gives rough estimate for parasitemia.
- **Thin blood film/smear:** Air dried for 10 minutes exposed to methanol.
- **Sensitivity:** 200 parasite/microlitre.
- It is specially useful for species identification and for exact quantification of Parasitemia.
- Stain used for Plasmodium is Romanowsky stain and Jaswant Singh Bhattacharya (JSB) stain.
- Quantitative Buffy Coat is method of identifying Plasmodium infected RBC's by the means of micro-centrifugation, fluorescence and density gradient.
- It has got highest sensitivity of 2 parasite/microlitre.

82. 66 years old man came to the OPD for his regular post transplant check up. Patient underwent Hepatic transplant due to cirrhosis 3 months ago. Since then he is on immunosuppressant like Tacrolimus and prednisolone. Consulting doctor noticed that patient's creatinine level have been increasing slowly but progressively since transplant. At the time of transplant his creatinine level was 1.0 mg/dL; after 1 month it was 1.3 mg/dL; after 2 months of transplant it was 1.55 mg/dL; currently after 3 months of transplant his creatinine level is 2.05 mg/dL. What is the cause of this creeping rise in creatinine and what can be the possible complication in this patient?

A. HHV-3; Chorioretinitis
B. BK virus; Post transplant nephropathy
C. JC virus; Liver graft failure/rejection
D. Mycobacterium; Renal TB

Answer: B. BK virus; Post transplant nephropathy

Solution

- This is the case BK virus associated post transplant nephropathy, which is characterised by creeping rise of creatinine.
- BK virus comes under category of polyoma virus.
- BK virus is ubiquitous infection.
- Whenever there is transplant the immunosuppressant can cause reactivation of BK virus that's present in latent form in kidney.
- One of the most pathognomic feature of BK virus reactivation is creeping slow rise of creatinine.
- There can be different signs and symptoms of BK virus at different stages of disease:
  1. Initially there is virurea followed by viremia.
  2. In urine there can be pyuria, microscopic hematuria and cast cell.
- One of most pathognomic findings of BK virus infection in urine analysis is presence of Decoy cells.

83. 62 years old male is admitted to the hospital with multiple neurological related complain: Progressive weakness, loss of coordination, worsening memory loss and homonymous hemianopia for last 2 days. He has fallen down twice while walking in last 2 days and his memory is worsening over time so much so that he can't even recognise her family members.There is no paralysis like symptoms noticed in patient. There is no history of trauma. Patient was recently diagnosed with non Hodgkin's lymphoma 2 months back and currently is on chemotherapy regime of Rituximab. There is no relevant family history. Upon physical examination it was not that patient pulse rate was 78, blood pressure of 126/88, respiratory rate of 20, oxygen saturation of 98% and fever was 100.8°C. Patient was oriented in time place but not in person.

At this stage consulting doctor conducted MRI of brain which showed multiple non enhancing lesion in areas of parietal lobe, occipital lobe and cerebellar lobe (image given below).

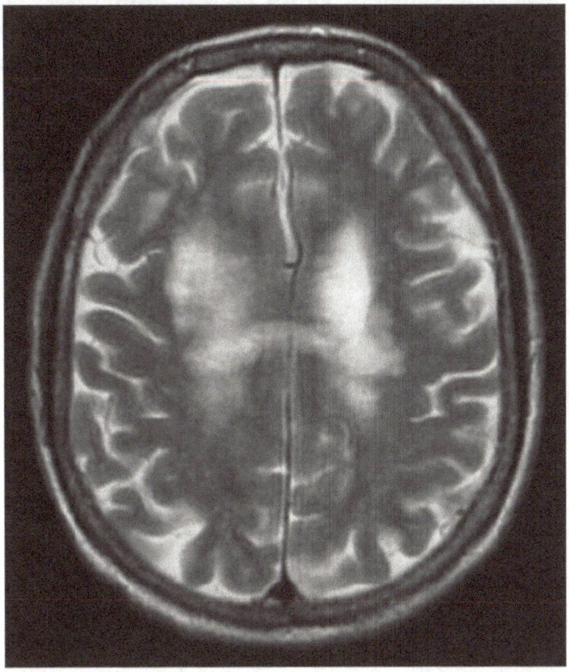

Source: Radswiki https://creativecommons.org/licenses/by-sa/3.0CC BY-SA 3.0 Creative Commons Attribution-ShareAlike 3.0

At this stage consulting doctor send serology for HIV, Japanese Encephalitis Virus, CMV, EBV and JC virus. Which later came out to be positive for IgM JC virus. Which of the following is correct regarding JC virus?

A. It comes under classification of Flavivirus

B. It is known to cause transplant nephropathy

C. It causes Progressive Multifocal Leukoencephalopathy which mainly affects Parietal lobe, occipital lobe and cerebellum

D. One of the pathognomic feature of JC virus is presence of decoy cell

Answer: C. It causes Progressive Multifocal Leukoencephalopathy which mainly affects Parietal lobe, Occipital lobe and cerebellum

Solution

- It is the case of reactivation of JC virus which comes under classification of Polyoma virus.
- JC virus is ubiquitous infection.
- It generally infects immunocompromised individual specially seen in individual who are on Rituximab and Natalizumab regime and HIV patients.
- HIV individual suffers from JC virus when CD count is less than 200.
- It is known to cause Progressive Multifocal Leukoencephalopathy: It has demyelinating effects on Parietal, Occipital and cerebellum areas of brain.

84. 5 years old girl was brought to OPD by her parents with multiple complain of fever (of 101°C) and malaise related symptoms for the last 6 days and also patient had difficulty in eating for the last 2 days. There is history of cough or chills. Patient has no associated recent travel history neither she has any history of being on contact with any patient at all. Child birth was uneventful occurred via normal vaginal delivery at 37 weeks of gestation. Her vaccine status is complete. On physical examination patient vitals were stable and she was oriented in time, place and person. On examination it was noted that she was having 2 peculiar papule on hand and foot each, similar papule were also noted on trunk (given in image below). Intra oral examination showed presence of multiple lesion (given in image below). At this stage your professor conducts serology for coxsackie virus and ask you which of the following is NOT correct regarding the pathogenic organism?

A. The given condition is mainly caused by group A of Coxsackievirus

B. Coxsackievirus is part of Enterovirus

C. They are classified under category of Flavivirus

D. It can also cause acute hemorrhagic conjunctivitis

Answer: C. They are classified under category of Flavivirus

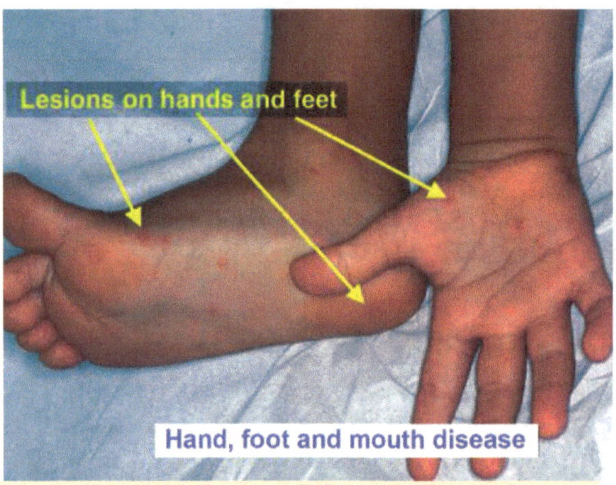

Source: Wikidoctor; Author: Usma Talib; License: Creative Common Attribution-ShareAlike 4.0 international license

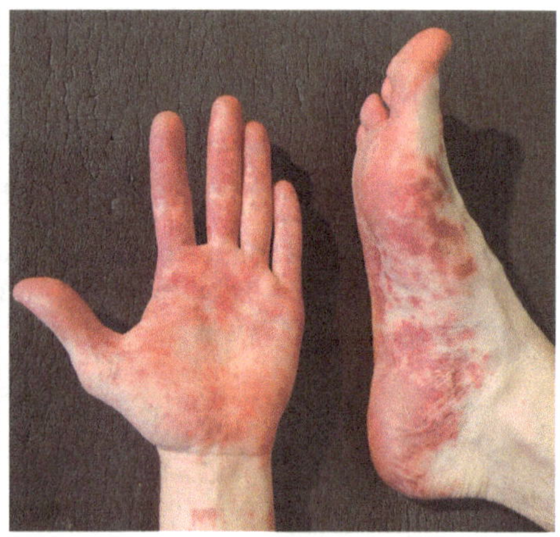

Source: Wikipedia; Author: VORONSPb, License: Creative Common Attribution-ShareAlike 4.0 International license

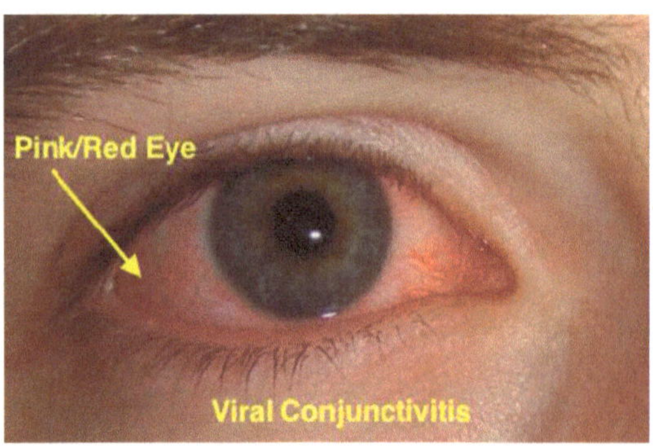

Source: Wikidoctor; Author: Usma Talib; License: Creative Common Attribution-ShareAlike 4.0 International license

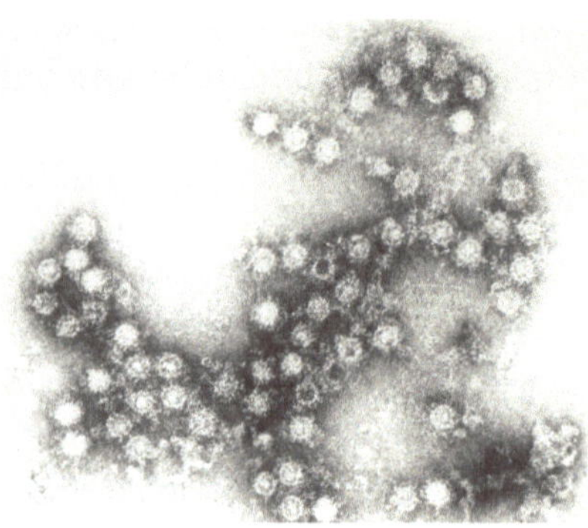

Coxsackievirus under immunoelectron microscope

Solution

- This is the case of hand, foot and mouth disease which is caused by Coxsackievirus.
- Coxsackievirus comes under classification of Enterovirus.
- Since Enterovirus are able to survive in pH of as low as 3. Hence they can resist and survive in low gastric pH.
- Therefore Mode of Transmission for Enterovirus is feco-oral route.
- Coxsackievirus is divided into two types on the basis of their pathogenicity in newborn suckling mice.
  1. Coxsackie A.
  2. Coxsackie B.
- **Incubation Period:** 2-9 days.
- Coxsackievirus can cause diverse clinical presentation and diverse types of syndrome.
- One of such disease caused by Coxsackievirus is 'Hand, foot and mouth syndrome'.
- It is caused by group A coxsackievirus.
- Mainly children are affected.
- There is characteristic rash on hand and feet along with ulcerative lesion in mouth.
- **Other Syndrome Caused by Coxsackie are:**
  1. **Herpangina:** Caused by group A coxsackievirus.
     - o Mainly affect children.
     - o It is characterised by fever, sore throat, anorexia, dysphagia, vomiting and abdominal pain.
  2. Self limiting disease.
  3. Pleurodynia.
  4. Myocarditis and Pericarditis.

85. 15 years old female comes to OPD with complain of sore throat, fever, cough and malaise related symptoms for the last 15 days. There is no related recent travel history. Patient is non smoker, non alcoholic with no known history of drug abuse. Patient's vaccine status is complete. Her menstrual cycle is regular and started since she was 13 years 10 months old. On physical examination her vitals were stable with pulse rate of 72/minute, Blood Pressure was 122/78, respiratory rate was 17/minute with oxygen saturation of 98%. She was oriented in time, place and person. There was no pallor on her face and neither there was any lesion examined on her body. Her neurological examination was unremarkable with no issue regarding vision. Based on this consulting doctor considered it to be normal case of bacterial pharyngitis and started patient on amoxicillin. 2 days later patient comes back with complain of maculopapular like lesion all over her body which probably occurred due to drug reaction. Based on this which of the following is NOT correct regarding pathogenic organism?

A. Primary site of Infection for pathogenic organism is Tonsils

B. Site of latency is B cell

C. Causative organism is known to cause Burkitt's lymphoma and Nasopharyngeal Carcinoma

D. It causes infectious mononucleosis like syndrome

E. On Complete Blood Count analysis we would notice presence of 'Downey cells'

Answer: D. It causes infectious mononucleosis like syndrome

Solution

- Based on clinical analysis it seems to be the case of infectious mononucleosis or kissing disease or glandular fever.
- It occurs due to HHV-4 or EBV (Epstein-Barr Virus).
- **Mode of Transmission:** Body fluids specially 'saliva'. Saliva remains the main source of infection since primary site of infection of EBV is Tonsils.
- HHV-4 enter B cell via CD-21 and CR-2 receptor and later cause Polyclonal proliferation of B cell eventually leading to carcinoma.
- EBV or HHV-4 is known to cause:
  1. Nasopharyngeal carcinoma.
  2. Burkitt lymphoma.
  3. Hodgkin or non-Hodgkin's lymphoma.
  4. Oral Hairy leukoplakia.
  5. Tonsillar carcinoma.
- EBV infects tonsils, enters B cell and undergoes latency evading the immune clearance system of our body.
- **Clinical Presentation of Infectious Mononucleosis:**
  1. Fever, chills and malaise related symptoms.
  2. Sore throat.
  3. Swollen lymph nodes.
  4. Swollen tonsils erythematous with white exudate.
  5. Carcinoma related complication can also occur.
  6. Interstitial pneumonia (in immunocompromised patients).

Diagnosis:

- On blood smear there is presence of 'Downey cells' or 'Atypical lymphocytes'.
- These are enlarged T lymphocytes with eccentric nuclei and vacuolated cytoplasm.
- One of the most peculiar characteristic of EBV is the presence of Heterophile antibody that are complement against 'Paul-Bunnell' antigen on sheep horse and bovine erythrocytes.
- Based on this we also conduct 'Paul Bunnell' test which is heterophile agglutination test.
- Also we can use PCR to detect certain antigens on EBV like Early antigen and Epstein-Barr Nuclear Antigen (EBNA).

Treatment:

- Currently there is no definitive treatment or preventive vaccine available for EBV.

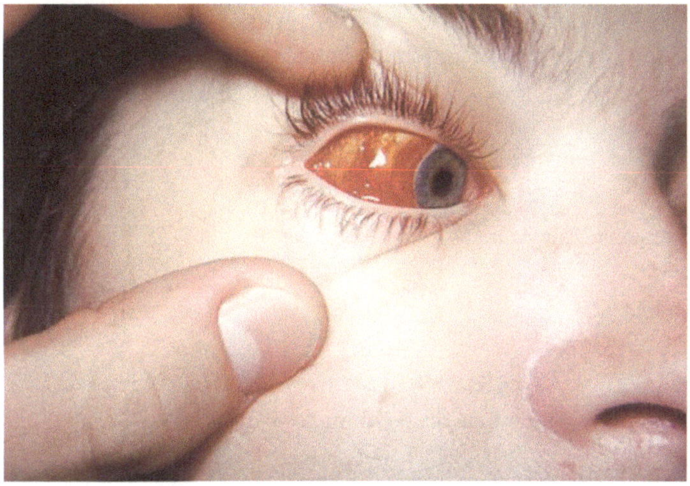

Conjunctival hemorrhage in patient of infectious mononucleosis

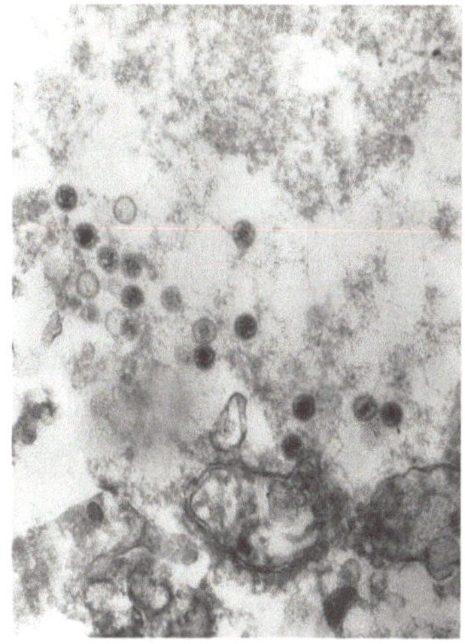

Transmission electron microscope showing EBV

86. 45 years old male comes with multiple complain of intermittent fever and malaise related symptoms along with progressive generalized weakness for the last 7 months. He has also been loosing weight for last 2 months, in last 2 months he has lost 15 kg. Patient is non alcoholic, non smoker with no known drug abuse. On physical examination patient looks dull.There was presence of generalised lymphadenopathy. There is no sign of icterus or any other sign of jaundice or hepatic disease. His vitals were pulse rate 90, Blood Pressure: 110/82, respiratory rate of 19/min. At this stage Complete Blood Count analysis was conducted which showed Pancytopenia, Hypergammaglobulinemia, no atypical cells were found. At this stage doctor decided to conduct bone marrow biopsy which showed following image of Leishmania donovani body in cytoplasm of macrophage.

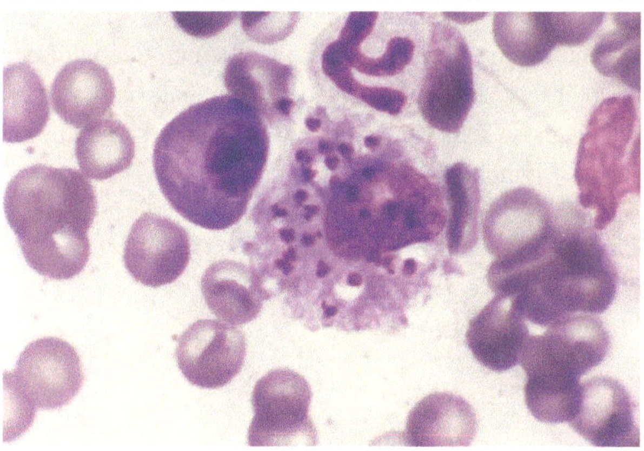

Which of the following is NOT correct regarding pathogenic organism?

A. Above mentioned condition is caused by Leishmania donovani complex (L. donovani, L. infantum, L. chagasi)

B. Vector is Phlebotomus argentipes

C. Site of latency is B-cell

D. Albumin: Globulin ratio is reversed

E. Confirmatory diagnosis can be done by doing ELISA for recombinant antigen rK-39

Answer: C. Site of latency is B-cell

Solution

- This is the case of Visceral leishmania/Kala azar.
- **Definitive Host:** Humans.
- **Habitat:** Reticuloendothelial cells.
- **Vector:** Sandfly.
- **Infective Form:** Promastigote.
- **Mode of Transmission:** Bite of sandfly, blood transfusion, through placenta.

Pathophysiology:

- Promastigote gets phagocytosed by Reticuloendothelial cells/macrophages and gets converted into amastigotes which undergoes binary fission and eventually causing the cell to rupture.
- If no immune response/antibody present then it again gets phagocytosed by macrophage and undergoes repeated cycles.

Clinical Features:

- **Incubation period** is of 3-5 months.
  1. Persistent intermittent fever.
  2. Progressive weight loss.
  3. Malaise related symptoms.

Diagnosis:

- Complete Blood Count analysis shows Pancytopenia (it occurs because Bone marrow contains proliferating macrophage containing amastigotes).
- Hypergammaglobulinemia causing reversible albumin: Globulin ratio.
- Best specimen to observe leishmania inside macrophage is not blood.
- To observe and diagnose Kala azar following specimen should be considered:
  - Bone marrow > lymph node.
- Under giemsa stain or leishmania stain we will be able to observe 'Leishmania donovani body' inside of macrophage which is actually kinetoplast or mitochondrial DNA of Leishmania.
- **Cultivation:** Novy–MacNeal–Nicolle medium.
- **Molecular Methods of Diagnosis:**
  - NAAT's.
  - ELISA for rK39 antigen.

Treatment:

- **Drug of Choice:**
  - Amphotericin B.
  - Oral miltefosine.
  - Antimony compound.
  - Sitamaquine.

87. 37 years old male presents to OPD with multiple complains of fever and malaise related symptoms for the last 7 days along with neck rigidity, photophobia and headache for the last 2 days. There is no associated visual anomaly. Patient has a 20 days travel history to Japan where he got involved in various activities like camping in rural side skydiving etc. He does give history of multiple mosquito bite during his visit. Patient is non smoker, alcoholic consume 1 can of beer every day, with no history of drug abuse. Patient's vitals were stable with Pulse rate 73, Blood Pressure of 138/88, respiratory rate of 22. On physical examination patient is oriented in time, place and person. No rash or lesion was spotted. Based on this doctor conducts Complete Blood Count analysis along with lumbar puncture which showed neutrophils 22% and lymphocytes 55% in blood. While CSF was clear, Glucose was more than ⅔rd of plasma glucose level and protein was minimally increased. At this stage consulting doctor send serology for EBV, mumps, measles, coxsackie, Enterovirus and Japanese Encephalitis Virus. Out of these IgM for Japanese Encephalitis Virus came out to be positive.

At this stage your professor ask you which of the following is NOT correct regarding this pathogenic organism?

A. Travellers are advised to be vaccinated before traveling to endemic areas

B. Vector-culex tritaeniorhynchus

C. Amplifying reservoir is pig

D. Ardeid (water) bird

E. Confirmatory diagnosis by blood culture

Answer: E. Confirmatory diagnosis by blood culture

Solution

- This is the case of Japanese Encephalitis Virus.
- **Epidemiology:** It is epidemic in East Asia.
- **Vector:** Culex tritaeniorhynchus.
- **Reservoir:** Ardeid birds.
- **Amplifying reservoir:** Pigs.

Clinical Presentation:

- **Incubation Period:** 5-15 days.
- **Symptoms:** Malaise related symptoms, fever, nausea, vomiting etc.
- **Later there is neurological manifestations like:** Meningitis, Cranial nerve palsy, speech abnormality, Parkinson like presentation and seizure.
- Mortality is 30%.
- Neurological sequelae in 50%.
- **Diagnosis:** Serology.
- **Confirmatory diagnosis:** PRNT (Plaque Reduction Neutralization Test).
- **Treatment** is symptomatic.
- Japanese Encephalitis Virus is part of Flavivirus.
- **Other Flaviviruses are:** West-Nile Virus, St. Louis encephalitis.

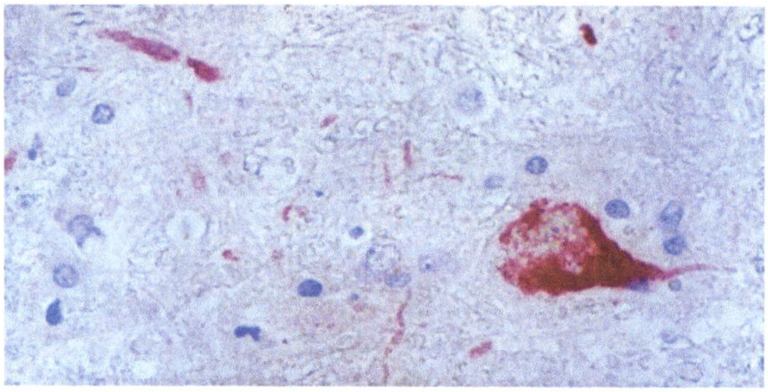

West-Nile virus in tissue specimen

88. 70 years old female was admitted to hospital with complain of fever, cough, dyspnea and other malaise related symptoms for the last 15 days. Patient has no associated travel history. Patient has medical history of controlled diabetes for the last 20 years and have been on metformin since then. On physical examination patient was oriented in time, place and person. Her vitals were slightly deranged with pulse rate 94, Blood Pressure of 145/92, respiratory rate of 25/minute, random glucose level was 145 mg/dL. Doctor conduct complete blood count which showed neutrophils 20% and lymphocytes 60%. Based on this consulting doctor conducts serology for CMV, EBV coxsackie, ECHO virus, influenza virus, adenovirus. Out of all of these IgM for influenza virus came out to be positive. At this stage your professor ask you which of the following is NOT correct regarding the pathogenic organism?

A. Only Influenza type A virus have variability of 'hemagglutinin' and 'Neuraminidase'

B. Anti neuraminidase antibody plays role in limiting disease

C. Antigenic shift is responsible for epidemics while Antigenic drift is responsible for pandemics

D. DOC is neuraminidase inhibitor like Oseltamivir, zanamivir

E. Antigenic shift is seen in Influenza A while Antigenic drift is seen in Influenza A, B and C

Answer: C. Antigenic shift is responsible for epidemics while Antigenic drift is responsible for pandemics

Solution

- This is the case of influenza virus that is part of Orthomyxovirus.
- Influenza virus is divided into 3 types on the basis of 'Matrix protein' and 'Ribonucleic protein'.
  1. **Influenza-A:** Causes pandemic and epidemic.
  2. **Influenza-B:** Causes epidemics.
  3. **Influenza-C:** Causes sporadic cases.
- Only Influenza type A shows hemagglutinin and neuraminidase variation.
- Lipid envelope of influenza virus contain 2 important glycoproteins:
  1. Hemagglutinin.
  2. Neuraminidase.
- Hemagglutinin is responsible for binding to 'Sialic Acid Receptor' present on respiratory epithelial cell mucosa and RBC's.

- Neuraminidase destroys Sialic acid Receptor and cause the release of virus in host cell.
- Therefore anti neuraminidase antibody plays a role in limiting spread of virus.
- There are total:
    1. 18 hemagglutinin subtypes.
    2. 11 neuraminidase subtypes.
- Neuraminidase and hemagglutinin shows 2 types of antigen variability:
    1. Antigenic shift.
    2. Antigenic drift.
- Antigenic shift is generally seen in Influenza type A and is responsible for pandemics.
- Generally it seems to occur once in every 10-12 years.
- Antigenic shift occurs when single cell is infected by 2 strains of influenza A virus.
- Antigenic drift occurs in Influenza type A, B and C and it is responsible for epidemics.
- Generally it seems to occur every 2-3 years.
- Antigenic drift occurs due to point mutation in viral DNA.
- **Clinical Presentation:**
    1. Fever.
    2. Cough chills.
    3. Myalgia.
    4. Malaise related symptoms.
    5. Pneumonia.
    6. Otitis media.
    7. Bronchiolitis.
- **Diagnosis:** Serology, ELISA.
- **Treatment: Drugs:** M2 ion.
- **Channel inhibitor:** Amantadine, Rimantadine.
- **Neuraminidase inhibitor:** Inhibit release of virus.

  Examples: Oseltamivir, Zanamivir.

89. 10 years old boy is admitted with complain of fever for the last 12 days along with stomach ache particularly in right upper quadrant for the last 3 days along with 5 episodes of vomiting in the last 3 days. He has no symptoms of cough or respiratory tract inflammation neither does he have any symptoms of jaundice or myalgia and arthralgia related symptoms. He has no known Drug allergy and his vaccination history is complete. On physical examination he looked sick with flushed face along with pallor. There is mild submandibular lymphadenopathy. His heart rate was increased probably due to fever. He had mild tenderness in right upper quadrant of stomach with no abdominal distension, guarding or rebound tenderness. His liver was mildly enlarged while spleen was of normal size. There were no petechial or hemorrhagic rashes on skin. He was oriented in time, place and person with no neurological or cardiovascular deficit. Doctor asks intern to collect peripheral blood for complete blood count following findings were noted hemoglobin level was 11.8, his peripheral blood smear showed normocytic and normochromix RBC's along with target cell, Basophillic stippling and banana crescent shaped gametocyte in normal sized RBC's.

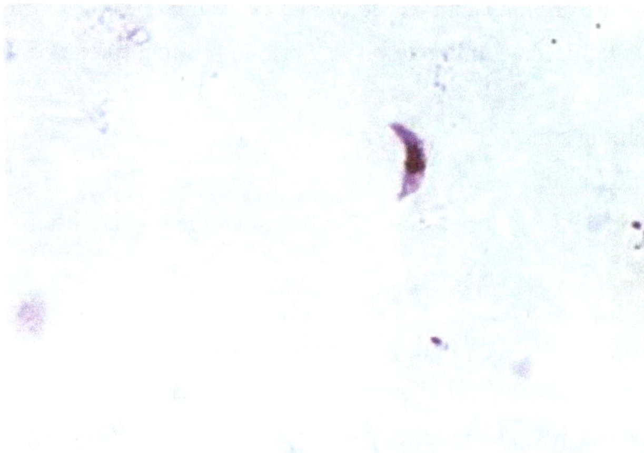

Banana/crescent shaped gametocyte

What is the pathogenic organism in this case?

A. Plasmodium falciparum

B. Clostridium

C. Nocardia

D. Corynebacterium

Answer: A. Plasmodium falciparum

Solution

- The given case is of malaria caused by Plasmodium.
- **Definitive host:** Female anopheles mosquito.
- **Intermediate host:** Human.

Clinical Features:

- Fever with chills, headache and malaise related symptoms.
- Mild anemia due to hemolysis, dyserythropoiesis, in severe cases there can be cerebral malaria + acute renal failure.
- Stains that we can use are Romanowsky stain or Jaswant Singh and Bhattacharya stain for plasmodium.

90. 45 years old female is brought to Emergency room with multiple complaints of fever and malaise related symptoms for the last 8 days; decrease urine output, shortness of breath and pedal edema for the last 2 days; confused, disoriented and 2 episodes of tonic clonic seizure since she woke up this morning. Patient has a recent travel history to Nigeria and have returned just 4 days ago. She is non smoker, non alcoholic with no history of drug abuse. Patient has uncontrolled Diabetic mellitus 2 for the last 14 years. She is not compliant with her drug intake. On physical examination there patient is oriented in place and person but not in time. There is mild icterus in eye. Pulmonary examination revealed presence of rattling sound while breathing. There is no rash or lesion on skin. Neither there is any sign of neck rigidity or photophobia. Doctor ask to conduct chest X-ray along with Total Blood Count study and Renal Function Test. Chest X-ray and Blood smear image is given below and RFT showed increased creatinine. What is incubation period of pathogenic species in this case?

A. 30 days
B. 12 days
C. 5 days
D. 20 days

Answer: B. 12 days

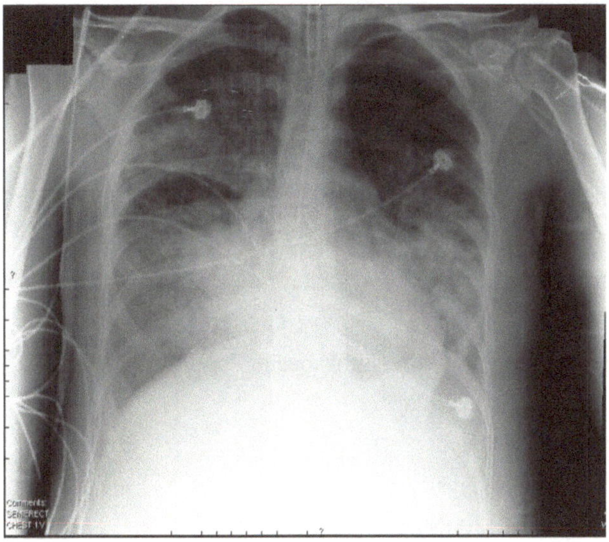

Chest X-ray

Source: File:Noncardiogenic pulmonary edema. JPG Author: Samir 04:51, 17 September 2007 (UTC) Permission (Reusing this file) Creative Commons Attribution-ShareAlike 3.0 Unported license

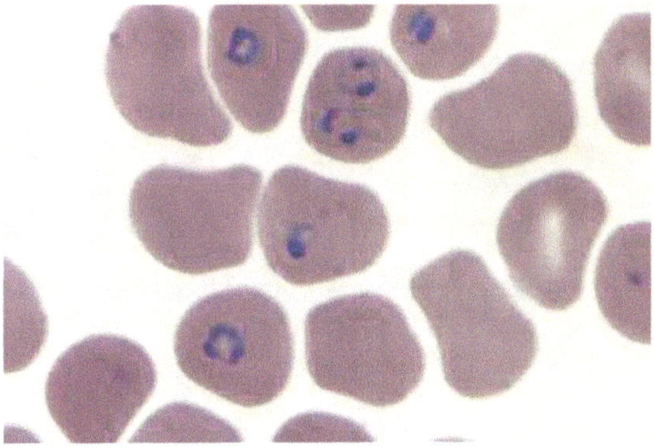

Blood smear

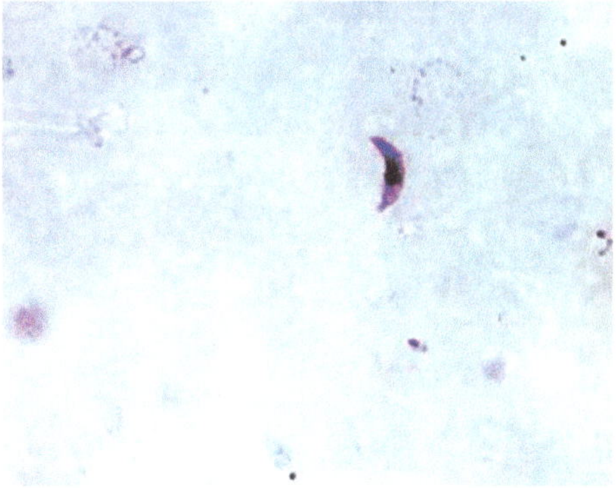

Blood smear

Solution

- This case is that of severe falciparum malaria caused by Plasmodium falciparum.
- The characteristic features of severe falciparum malaria is cerebral malaria along with acute renal failure.
- In cerebral malaria there can be seizure, confusion, disorientation.
- In acute renal failure there can be pedal edema, pneumoniae, shortness of breath etc.
- The incubation period in plasmodium is 1 Liver cycle + 2-3 RBC cycle.

- Severe falciparum malaria occurs due to sequestration of infected RBC's into the narrow arteries resulting into the complications like acute renal failure.
- There are 3 stages that lead to severe falciparum malariae:
    1. **Cytoadherance:** It is the property of plasmodium infected RBC's to adhere to the endothelial cells leading to narrowing of lumen.
    2. **Rosetting:** Binding of unparasitic RBC to parasite infected RBC.
    3. **Agglutination:** Binding of RBC's together.
- There are 5 types of Plasmodium species:
    1. Plasmodium falciparum.
    2. Plasmodium ovale.
    3. Plasmodium vivax.
    4. Plasmodium knowlesi.
    5. Plasmodium malariae.
- Incubation period of different plasmodium species:
    1. Plasmodium falciparum: 12 days.
    2. Plasmodium ovale: 14 days.
    3. Plasmodium vivax: 14 days.
    4. Plasmodium malariae: 30 days.
    5. Plasmodium knowlesi: 11 days.

Different characteristic appearances of different species of plasmodium:

Plasmodium Falciparum

- Normal sized RBC's with single or multiple rings early trophozoites.
- Accole or oblique forms of early trophozoites.
- Banana/crescent shaped gametocyte.

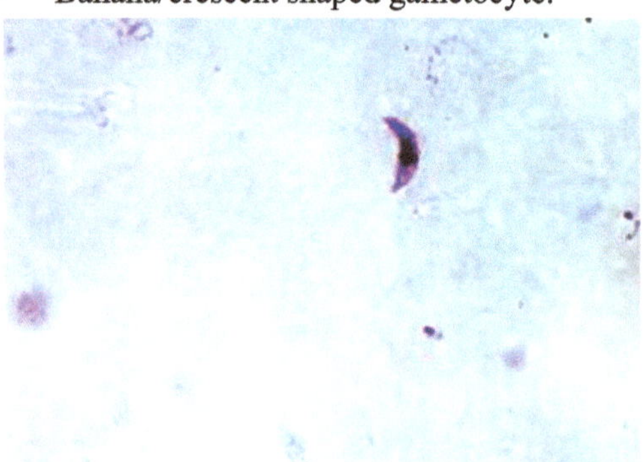

Banana or crescent shaped gametocyte

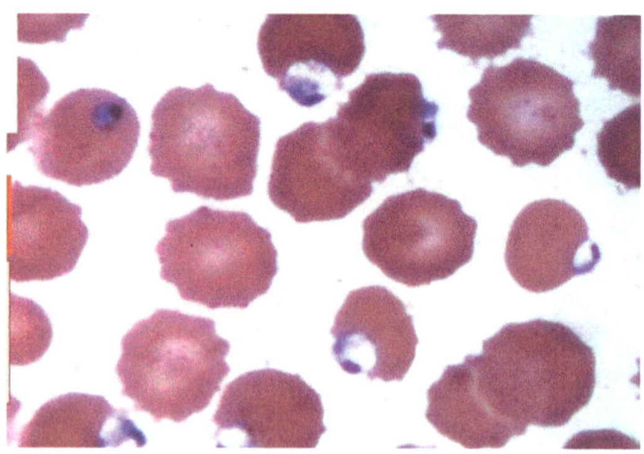

Accole or applique form of early trophozoites

Plasmodium Vivax

- Single ringed early trophozoites.
- Enlarged RBC's.
- Late trophozoites.
- Schizont.

- Amoeboid gametocyte.

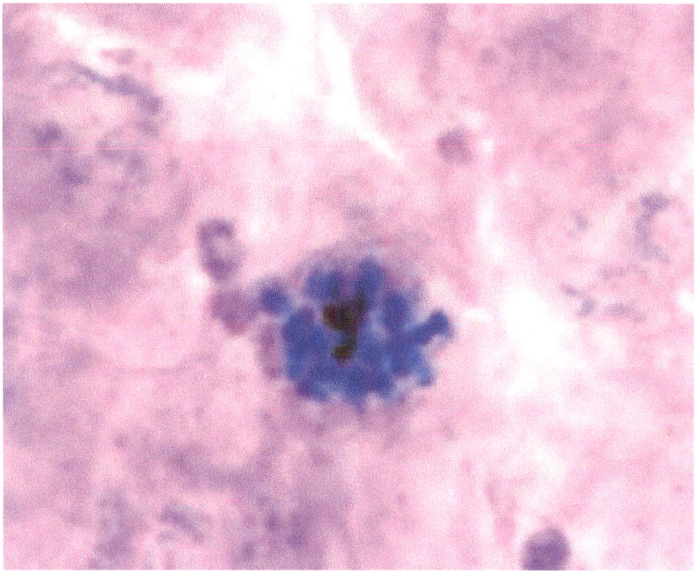

Schizont of P. vivax in a thick blood smear

Plasmodium Ovale

- Single ring early trophozoites.
- Old trophozoites.
- Schizont.
- Amoeboid gametocyte.
- Enlarged RBC's.

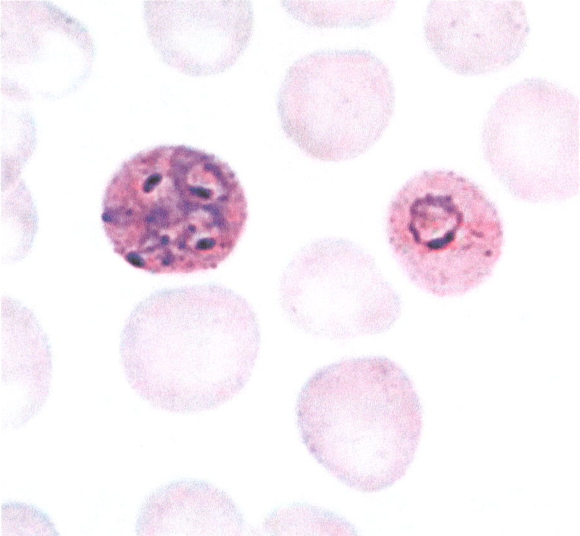

Ring-form trophozoites of P. ovale in a thin blood smear

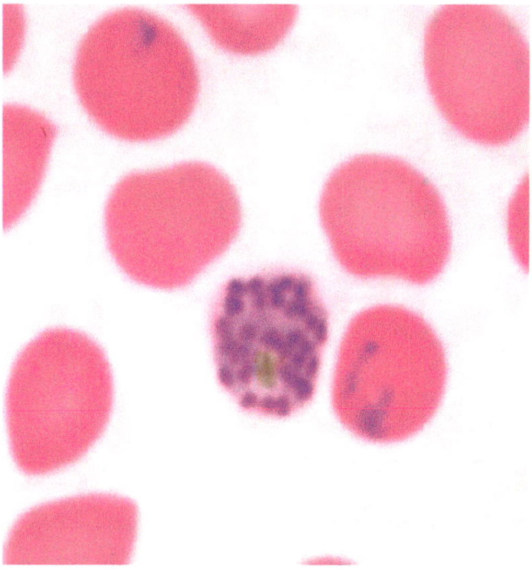

Schizont and amoeboid gametocyte

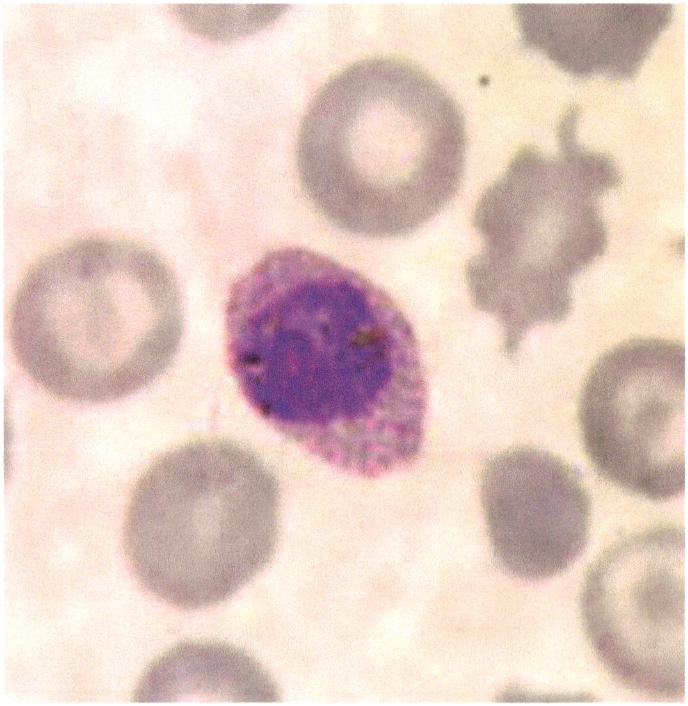

Trophozoite of P. ovale in a thin blood smear

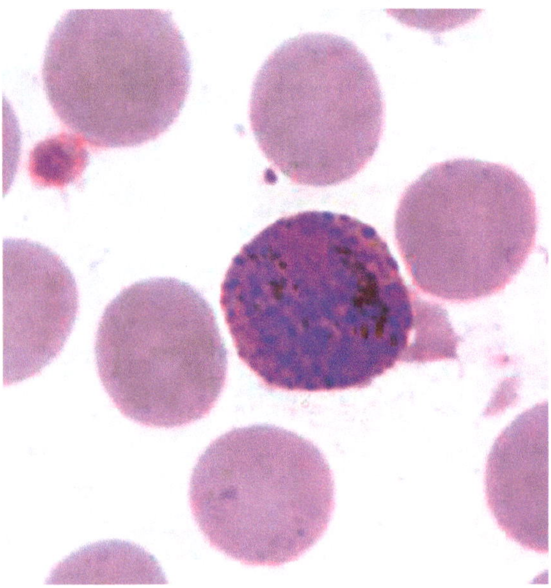

Macrogametocyte of P. ovale in a thin blood smear

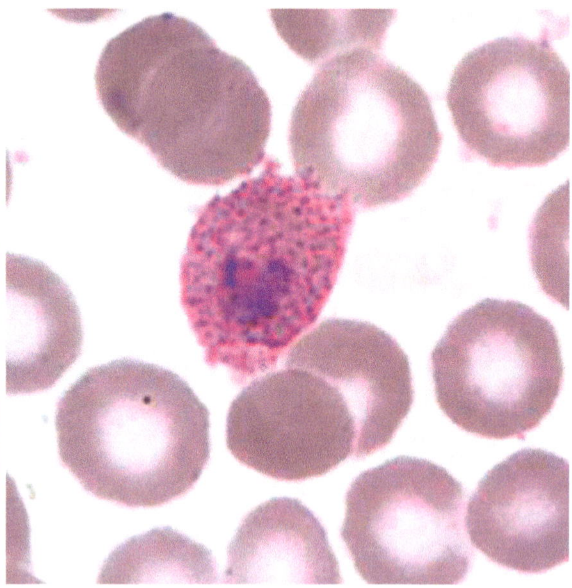

Microgametocyte of P. ovale in a thin blood smear

Plasmodium Malariae

- Normal sized RBC's with single ring early trophozoites.
- Schizont.
- Amoeboid gametocyte.

- Band-form of late trophozoites.

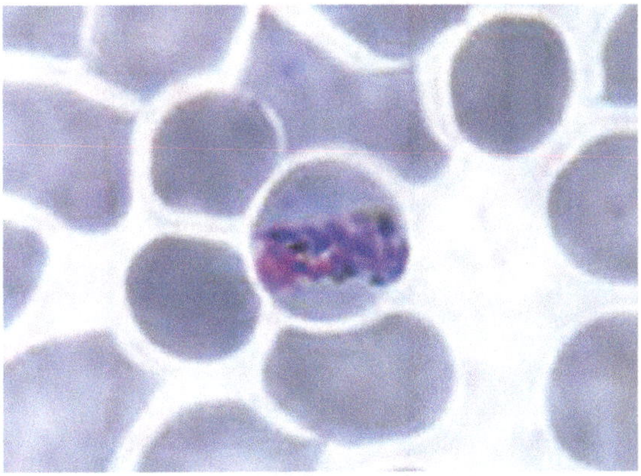

Band-form of trophozoites of Plasmodium malariae

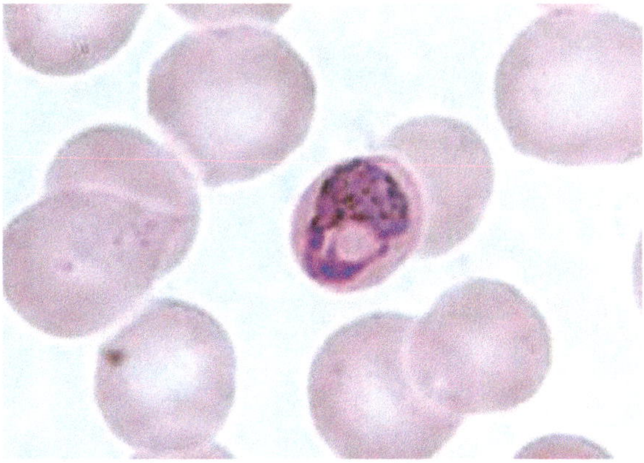

Basket-form trophozoite of P. malariae in a thin blood smear

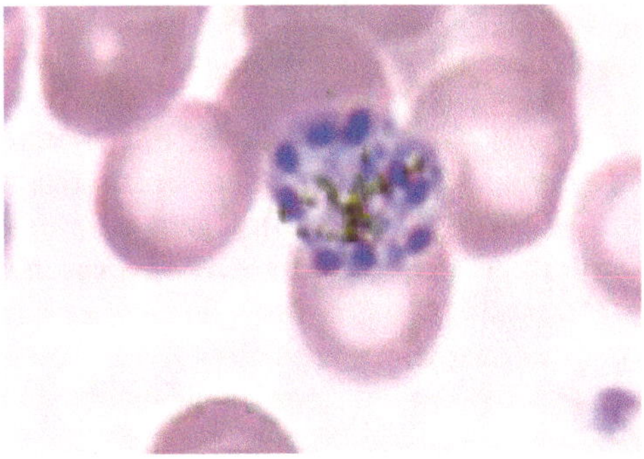

Schizont of P. malariae in a thin blood smear

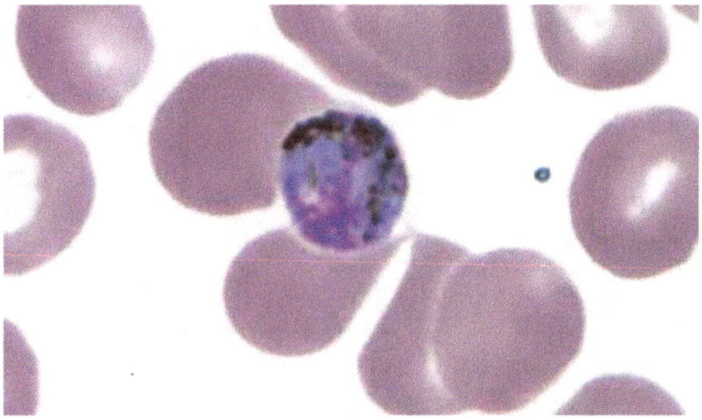

Gametocyte of P. malariae in a thin blood smear

Plasmodium Knowlesi

- Its blood smear has both Plasmodium malariae and falciparum characteristic cells.

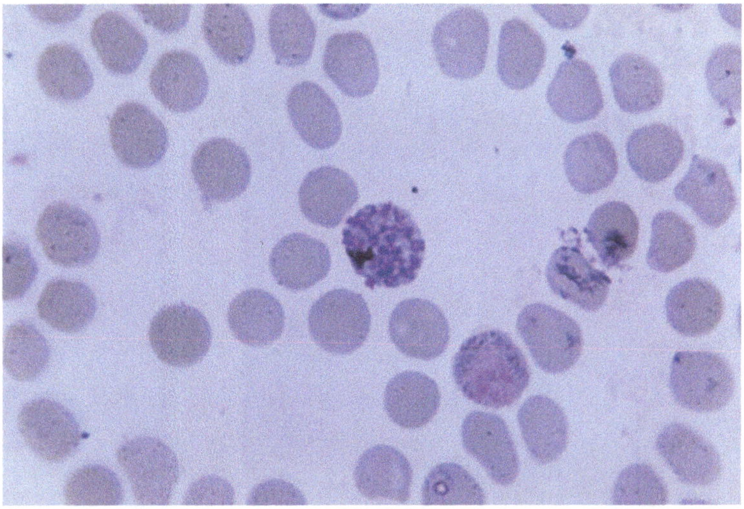

Under a magnification of 1125X, this photomicrograph of a simian blood sample revealed the presence of a mature, simian malarial schizont and gametocyte

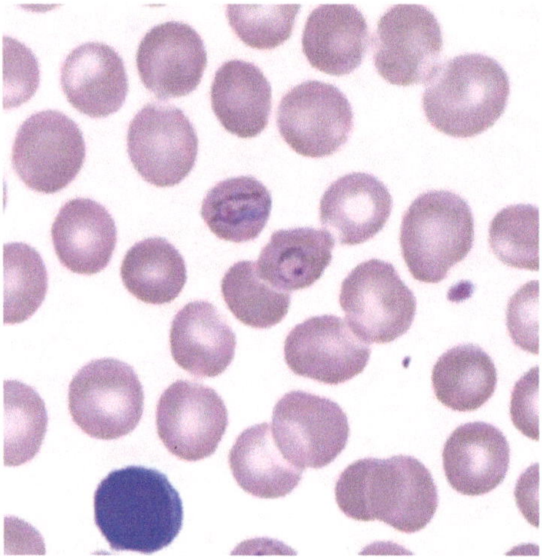

Band-form (upper) and ring-form (lower) trophozoites of P. knowlesi

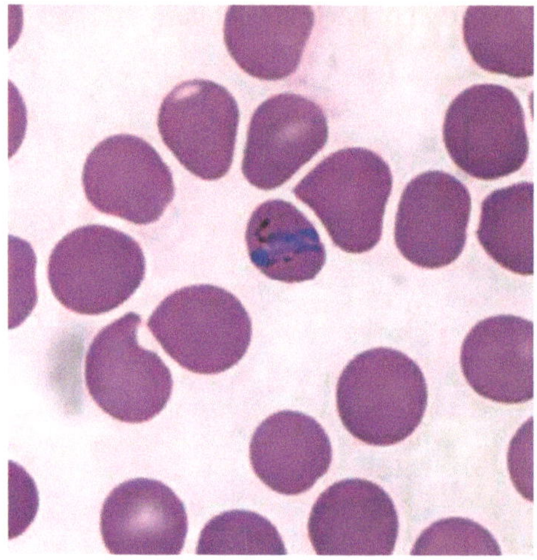

Band-form trophozoite of P. knowlesi in a Giemsa-stained thin blood smear

91. 35 years old female gave birth at 35 weeks of gestation via C-section. Newborn had microcephaly, bulging fontanelles, prominent scalp vein. On ophthalmic examination 'Chorioretinitis' was noted. Mother of the child was severely infected with COVID-19 during first trimester of her pregnancy and was on steroids for 2 weeks in self quarantined at home. Mother had a cat in her house and was in constant exposure to cat fecal matter. On conducting CT scan of head of newborn there were multiple Intracerebral calcification. Doctor was suspicious regarding transplacental opportunistic Infection occurring during first trimester of pregnancy and send newborn blood for giemsa staining and results are shown below in image.

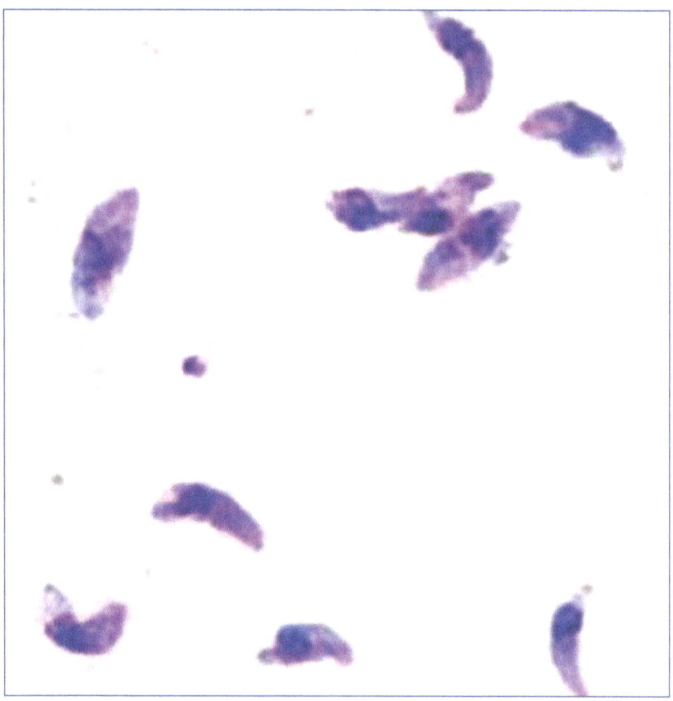

On conducting serology test of mother's blood IgM was negative while IgG was found to be positive. Also IgG was high in avidity. What is the Drug of choice for mother and newborn?

A. No treatment is required for mother for congenital toxoplasmosis; give Pyrimethamine + sulphadiazine + folinic acid for 1 year

B. Both mother and child should be given Pyrimethamine + sulphadiazine + folinic acid for 4 weeks

C. Both mother and child should be given Pyrimethamine + sulphadiazine + folinic acid for 6 months

D. Mother and child should be given Pyrimethamine + sulphadiazine + folinic acid for 1 year

Answer: A. No treatment is required for mother for congenital toxoplasmosis; give Pyrimethamine + sulphadiazine + folinic acid for 1 year

Solution

- This case is of congenital toxoplasmosis.
- Symptoms of congenital toxoplasmosis:
    - o Microcephaly.
    - o Hydrocephaly.
    - o Convulsions.
    - o Intracerebral calcification.
    - o Chorioretinitis.
- Congenital toxoplasmosis is caused by Toxoplasma.
- Definitive host of toxoplasma–Cats.
- Intermediate host of toxoplasma–Rodents, sheep, pigs.
- Humans are dead end host.
- **Infective form:** Sporulated cyst.
- **Mode of Infection:** Humans can get Sporulated cyst by contaminated food and water or by getting exposed to cat fecal matter or during gardening.
- Generally Toxoplasma do not infect immunocompetent individuals.
- If immunocompetent individual gets infected it is usually fever, malaise, headache and lymphadenopathy which resolve spontaneously no need of any intervention.
- It is called 'Infectious Mononucleosis like syndrome'.
- In immunosuppressants individual there can be symptoms like:
    - o *Encephalitis:* Causing altered mental status, seizures, nerve palsy, motor and sensory deficit.
    - o Pneumocystic pneumonia.

Diagnosis:

- Giemsa staining for diagnosing Tachyzoites in CSF or blood specimen.
- Direct fluorescent Antibody testing.
- Serology.
- PCR for blood and CSF for B 1 gene.

Treatment:

- For immunosuppressants individual–Pyrimethamine + Sulphadiazine + Folinic acid for 6 weeks.
- For congenital toxoplasmosis–Pyrimethamine + sulphadiazine + folinic acid.

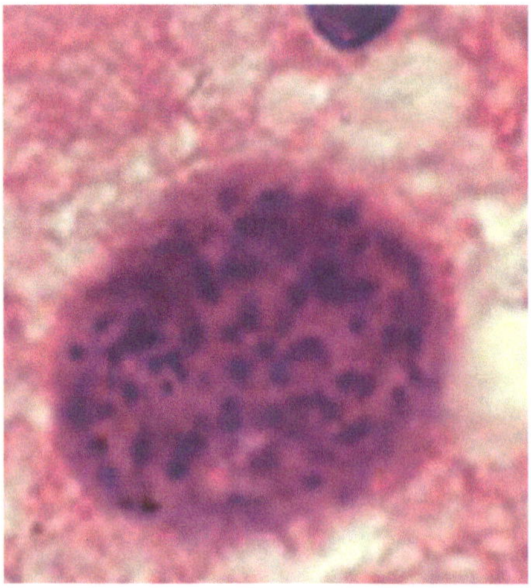

Toxoplasma gondii cyst in brain tissue

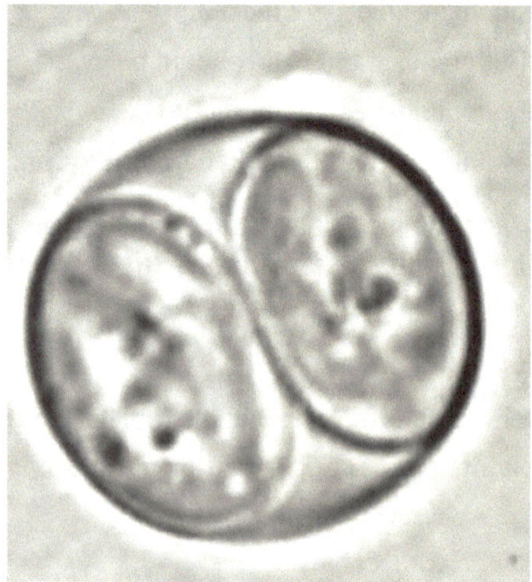

Toxoplasma gondii sporulated oocyst in an unstained wet mount

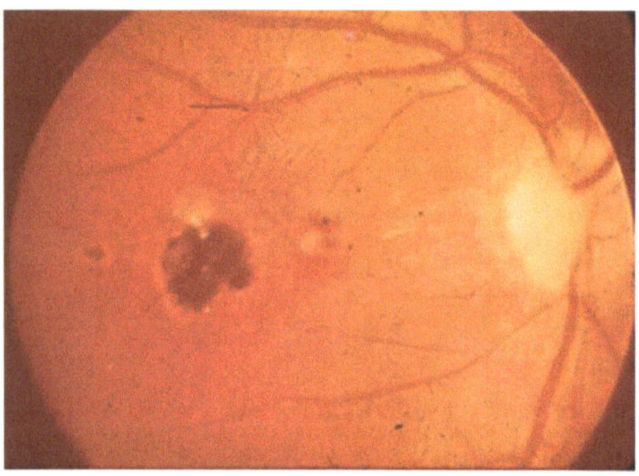

Central, healed retinochoroiditis

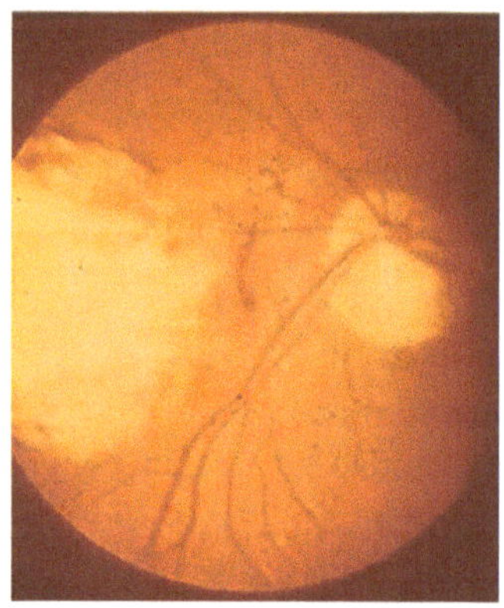

Severe, active retinochoroiditis

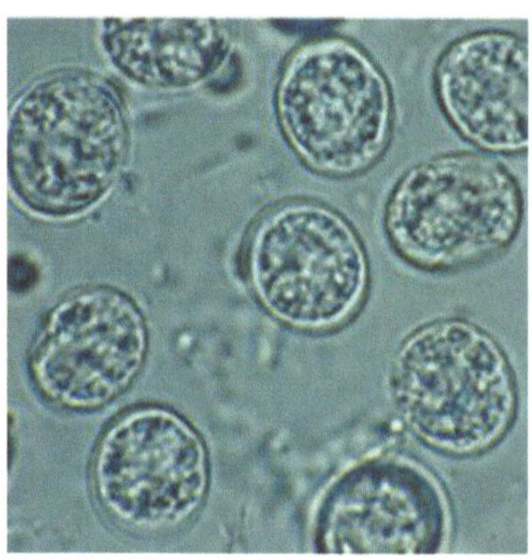

T. gondii oocysts in a fecal floatation

92. 25 years old male presented to OPD after he noticed hematuria in his first voiding of the day. Patient is non smoker, non alcoholic with no family history of squamous cell carcinoma of bladder. There is no history of recent infection but he does give history of him having mild urgency and burning pain upon micturition for the last 15 days. Based on this symptoms and history patient asks intern to conduct Ultrasound (KUB) along with urine analysis which showed calcification of bladder and urine analysis given below:

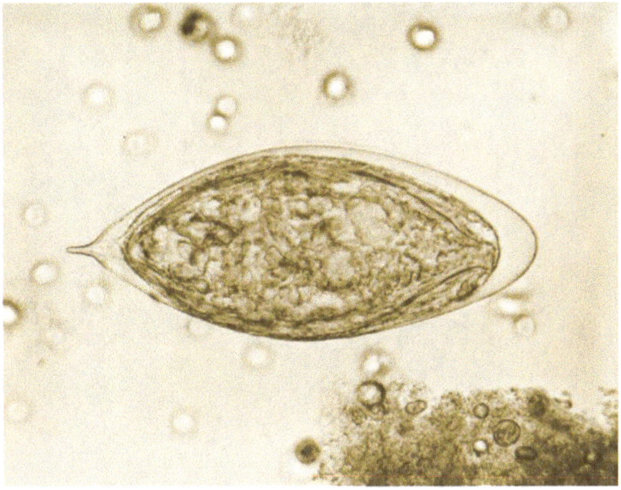

Where does pathogenic organism is normally resides in our body?

A. Inferior mesenteric plexus

B. Superior mesenteric plexus

C. Vesical plexus

Answer: C. Vesical plexus

Solution

- The given case is that of urine Infection caused by Schistosomiasis haematobium (its egg is non operculated domain with terminal spine).
- **Definitive host:** Mammals.
- **2 intermediate host:** First – Snail/molluscs.
  Second – Fresh water fish/plant.
- **Infective form:** Metacercariae.
- **Mode of Infection:** Consumption of fresh water fish infected with Metacercariae.
- Schistosomiasis haematobium causes SCC of bladder, Urinary Tract Infection, hydroureter, cercarial dermatitis (swimmers itch).
- It also causes calcification of urinary tract.
- Schistosomiasis haematobium resides in vesical plexus.
- Schistosomiasis mansoni resides in inferior mesenteric plexus.
- Schistosomiasis japonicum resides in superior mesenteric plexus.
- **Drug of Choice:** Praziquantel.

93. 40 years old male comes with multiple complains of diarrhea and abdominal pain for the last 17 days (3 motions in a day) which later turned into bloody diarrhea for the last 2 days, blood in vomit for the last 2 days, melena for the last 2 days. Patient is non smoker, non alcoholic or drug abuse. Patient has recent history of travel to Egypt for holiday. Patient has no history of jaundice. Upon general examination it was noted that patient had splenomegaly with no hepatomegaly. Patient have no pigmentation on skin. Attending doctor sends stool specimen for analysis which showed following findings.

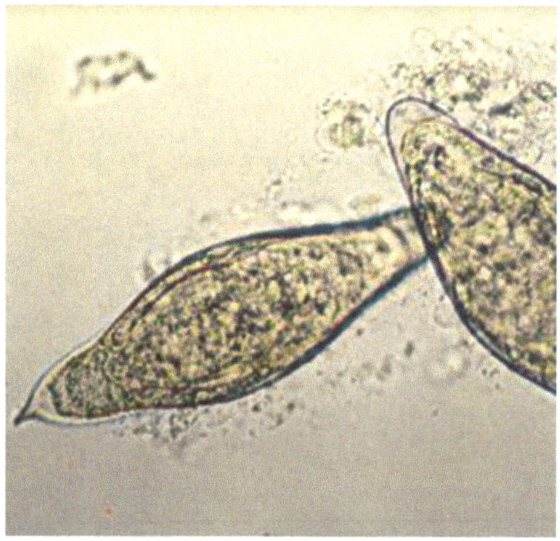

What is the Drug of Choice for this case?

A. Pyrimethamine
B. Sulphadiazine
C. Praziquantel
D. Folinic acid

Answer: C. Praziquantel

Solution

- The given case is that of Katayama fever caused by Schistosoma mansoni or Schistosoma intercalutum.
- **Definitive host:** Mammals.
- **2 Intermediate host:**
  - o First–Snails and mollusc.
  - o Second–Fresh water plant or fresh water fish.
- **Infective form:** Metacercariae.
- **Mode of infection:** Ingestion of fish with Metacercariae.
- **Different types of eggs of different schistosoma:**
  1. *Schistosoma haematobium:* Non operculated egg with terminal spine.
  2. *Schistosoma mansoni or intercalutum:* Non operculated egg with lateral spine.
  3. *Schistosoma japonicum:* Non operculated or sub spherical or oval with terminal knob.

- **Symptoms of Katayama disease:** Abdominal pain, bloody diarrhea and Portal hypertension.
- **Diagnosis:** Serology ELISA FAST (Falcon Assay Screening Test).
- **Drug of Choice:** Praziquantel.

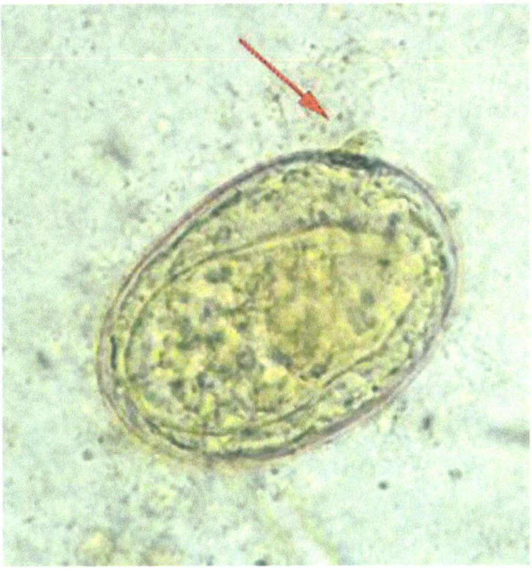

Egg of S. japonicum

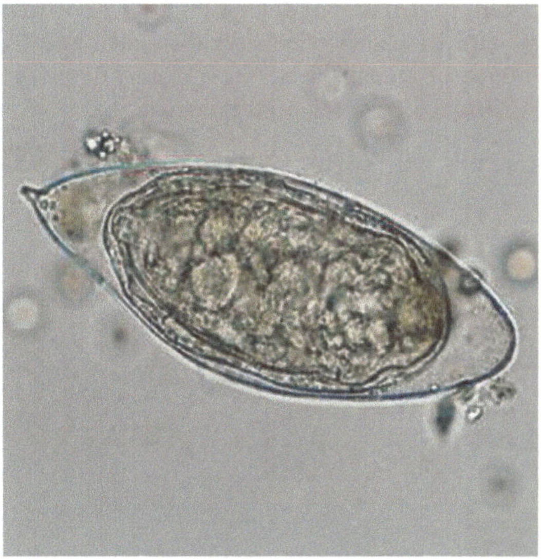

Egg of S. haematobium

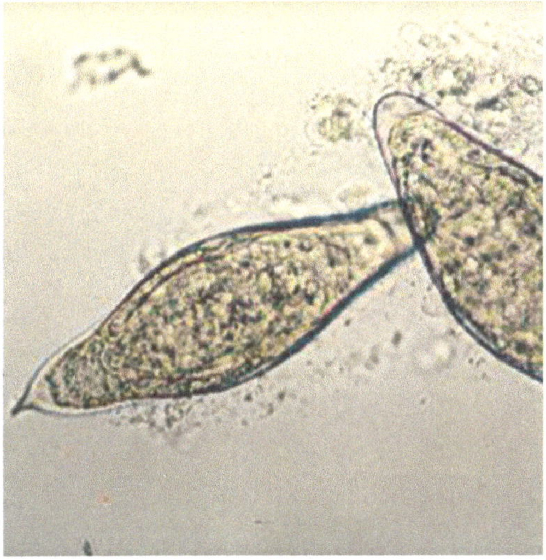

Egg of S. intercalatum

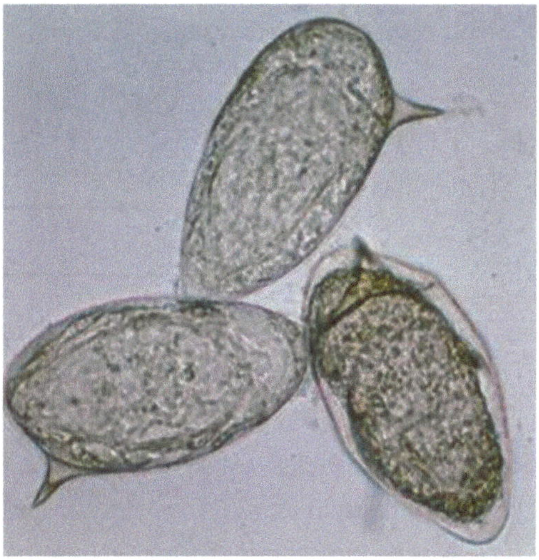

Egg of S. mansoni

94. 39 years old male comes with multiple complain of abdominal pain, bloating, alternating diarrhea and constipation for the last 16 days along with complain of mild fever, progressive dyspnea for the last 2 days. There is no history of blood in stools. 4 months ago patient was diagnosed with pulmonary TB for which he is currently on 6 months regime of Rifampicin and Isoniazid. Patient is gardner and has a history of working in garden bare footed. There is no associated travel history. Patient is a non smoker, non alcoholic with no history of drug abuse. He has been

following his normal dietary pattern. On physical examination his vitals were pulse rate: 91, blood pressure: 155/92, respiratory rate: 25, fever: 101.1°C, oxygen saturation was 86%. On examining the patient it was found that patient had presence of petechial skin lesion on foot along with vesicular eruption on thigh and buttock. On abdominal examination his abdomen was soft centrally tender, markedly distended and bowel sound were sluggish. Based on this consulting doctor conducts chest X-ray and Complete Blood Count which showed consolidation and high Eosinophils. Based on this doctor send stool sample which showed the following image.

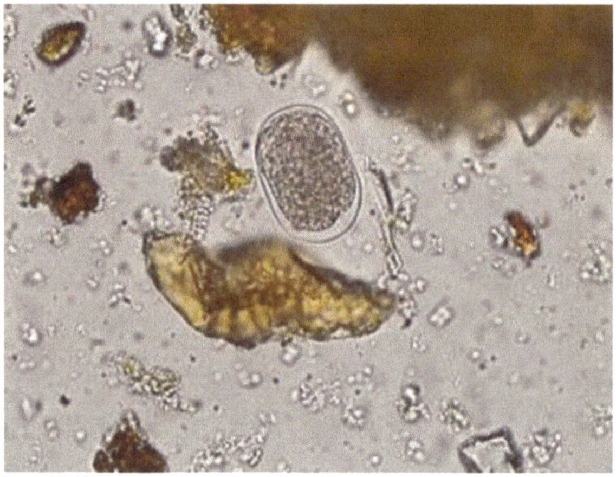

What is the drug of choice for this patient?

A. Acyclovir
B. Ivermectin
C. Ampicillin
D. Praziquantel
E. Pyrimethamine

Answer: B. Ivermectin

Solution

- This is the case of Strongyloides stercoralis infection.
- It is classified under intestinal nematodes.
- Generally found free living in soil.
- **Habitat in human:** Duodenum and upper jejunum.
- **Mode of infection:** Penetration by skin (Hence in this case since there is history of patient working bare footed in soil making him prone for this infection).
- **Infective form:** Filariform larva.

Clinical Features:

1. Petechial painful skin lesion at site of entry (in this case foot as given in image).
2. Vesicular eruption in area of thigh and buttock due to autoinfection by parasite in stool (Larva currents) (as given in question and shown in image).
3. **Loefflers syndrome:** Larvae in lungs causing Pneumonia (this is the cause for dyspnea and consolidation in lungs).

4. It can also cause abdominal bloating.
5. Malabsorption can also be there.
6. Alternating diarrhea and constipation.

Diagnosis:

- Specimen like sputum, stool, duodenal aspirate showed presence of Rhabditiform larvae in lugol or iodine stain.
- **Serology:** ELISA, Luciferase immunoprecipitation assay.
- **PCR.**
- **Drug of Choice:** Ivermectin for 2 days.
- There can also be disseminated strongyloidiasis which manifest as Gram-negative septicaemia, Meningitis and brain abscess.
- **Risk Factors for Disseminated Strongyloidiasis:**
  1. AIDS.
  2. Glucocorticoid therapy.
  3. Transplant.
- **Drug of Choice:** Ivermectin for 2 weeks.

95. 35 years old male comes to ER with primary complain of abdominal pain for the last 36 hours. Pain is continuous, progressive and cramping in nature. It started as mild cramping pain but over time became unbearable in umbilical region of stomach. Patient had no bowel movement for the last 3 days. Patient gives a history that he is feeling bloating in abdomen. There is no history of vomiting or nausea, neither there is any history of blood in stools. There is no associated recent travel history and patient have mainly stuck to his usual day-to-day diet. Patient is non smoker, non alcoholic with no history of drug abuse. Patient is normotensive and non diabetic. On physical examination patient vitals are stable with slightly raised Pulse rate of 83 (probably due to pain), Blood Pressure of 140/88, Respiratory Rate of 17/min and normal temperature. On abdominal examination, the shape of abdomen is round and bloating, on auscultation frequency of peristalsis sound is increased, palpation abdomen was tender with no hepatomegaly or splenomegaly, on percussion dull note was heard over hepatic, splenic area and resonance sound was heard over bowel area.

At this stage patient was taken for immediate open laparotomy. During laparotomy worm was extracted which was responsible for volvulus. Which of the following is NOT correct regarding pathogenic organism?

A. Mode of infection: Ingestion of egg with Rhabditiform larva
B. Can cause Loeffler syndrome with patchy round infiltrate in lungs
C. Also called restless wanderers
D. Diagnosis can be made by stool, sputum examination which shows presence of egg
E. Drug of choice is Albendazole

Answer: D. Diagnosis can be made by stool, sputum examination which shows presence of egg

Solution

- This is the case of ascaris infection causing complications of volvulus.
- Ascaris comes under classification of Intestinal Nematode.
- Other species of Intestinal Nematode are:
  1. Strongyloides stercoralis.
  2. Hookworm or ancylostoma.
- Ascaris is also called Restless wanderers as they can freely wander around in our body and can even come out of nose, mouth or anal cavity.
- **Habitat of ascaris:** Jejunum.
- **Mode of Transmission:** Ingestion of egg with Rhabditiform larva.

Clinical Features:

1. **Large Intestine related:** Obstruction, volvulus, intussusception and in severe cases perforation.
2. They can cause Loeffler syndrome they migrate to pulmonary region causing fever, dry cough, dyspnea and on X-ray there will be round patchy infiltrate.
3. **Malnutrition:** Vitamin A deficiency.
4. Appendicitis.
5. Pancreatitis.

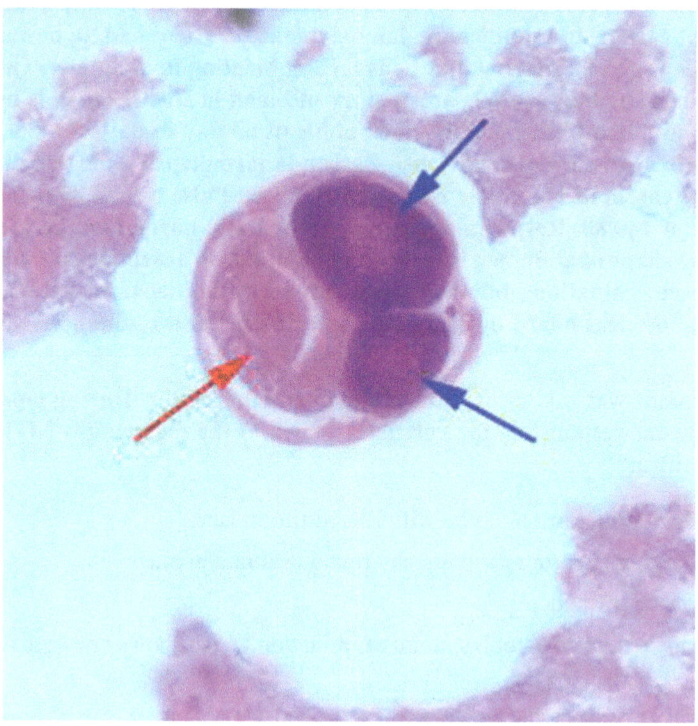

Schistosoma stercoralis stained present in small intestine

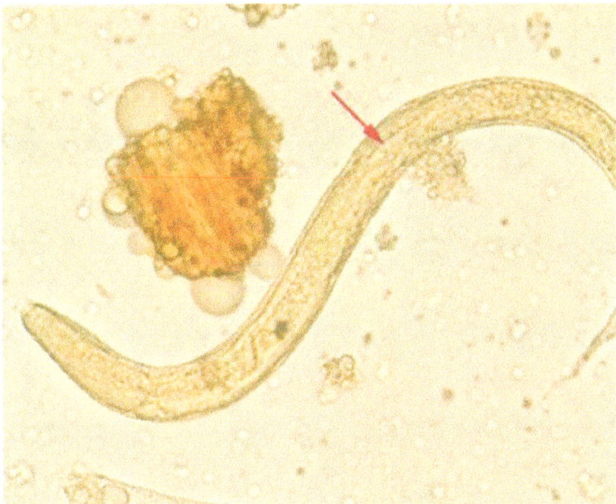

Rhabditiform larva of Schistosoma stercoralis shown in wet mount of stool

Diagnosis:

- Stools examination shows presence of egg of ascaris.
- Sputum analysis is only positive in transpulmonary stage and will show Filariform larvae.

Treatment:

- **Drug of Choice:** Albendazole.

96. 40 years old male comes with primary complain of abdominal pain continuous and dull over right hypochondrial region for the last 7 days. Patient is having normal bowel movement. Pain is not associated with food intake. There is no history of constipation or diarrhea. There is no history of vomiting or nausea neither there is any history of blood per rectum. There is no associated recent travel history. There is no history of any hepatitis infection or jaundice. Patient has remained on his usual diet. Patient is non alcoholic, non smoker with no known history of drug abuse.Patient has hypertension for the last 5 years and is well under control by ACE inhibitor. There is no family history related to hepatic cancer. There is no other remarkable personal history or medical history or family history.

On physical examination patient has BMI of 20.8 and his vitals are stable with pulse rate of 72, blood pressure of 122/78, respiratory rate of 19 and normal temperature. There are no signs of icterus in eye. There are no peculiar lesion or rash to be found on body. On abdominal examination abdomen was of normal shape flat, on auscultation only normal peristaltic sound at normal frequency were heard, on percussion normal dull note was heard at hepatic and splenic region along with resonating sound heard in bowel region, on palpation hepatomegaly was detected. Based on this hepatic ultrasound was conducted which showed the presence of multiple hypoechoic lesion. On conducting complete blood count analysis increased levels of Eosinophils were found. Later ultrasound guided fine needle biopsy was performed which showed presence of eosinophilic granuloma and parasite with help of special stain. What is the most probable diagnosis of given case?

A. Hepatic Cellular Carcinoma

B. Visceral larva migrans

C. Larva currens

D. Fitz Hugh Curtis Syndrome

Answer: B. Visceral larva migrans

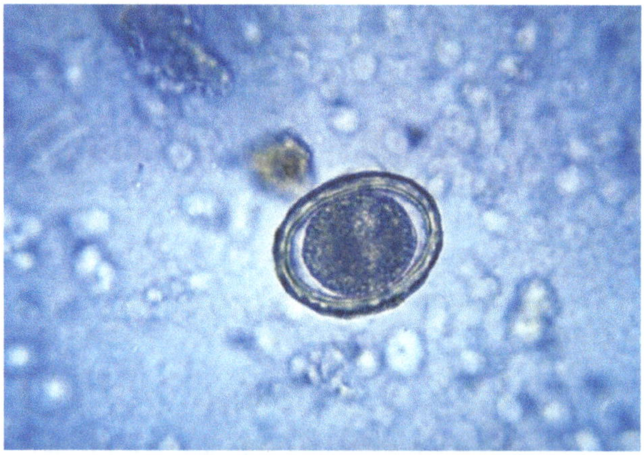

Egg of Ascaris lumbricoides

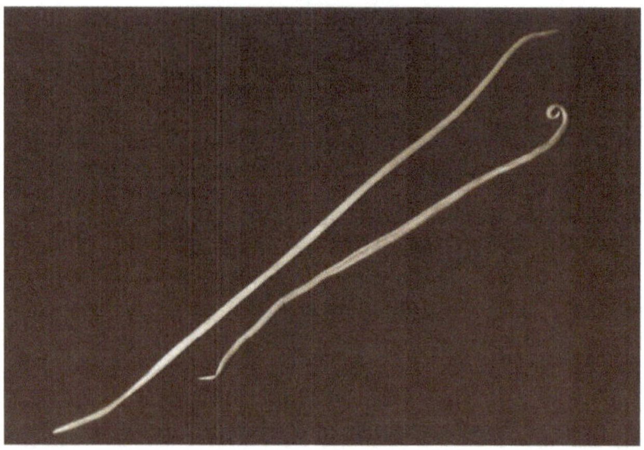

Ascaris

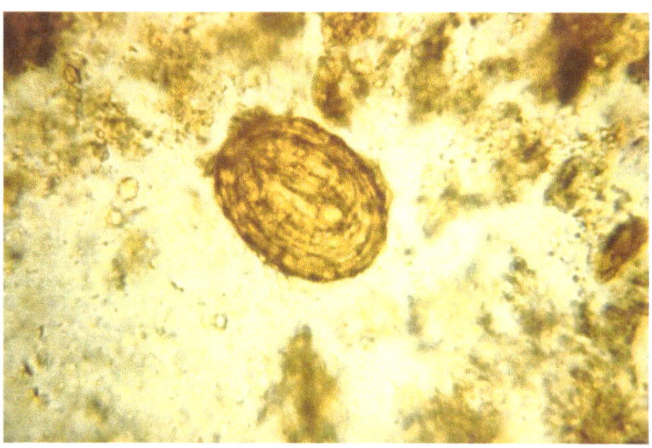

Egg of Ascaris lumbricoides

97. 21 years old male admitted due to watery diarrhea and dehydration for the last 20 days. There is no history of blood in stool, there is no associated history of nausea or vomiting or any abdominal pain. Patient is a university student. Patient is non alcoholic, non smoker with no history of drug abuse. Patient has no recent travel history but he has a history of playing football bare footed in an open field near his college. He has been on his regular dietary pattern. On physical examination patient vitals were stable with mild fever of 100.4, pulse rate 72, blood pressure: 133/82, oxygen saturation 98%, respiratory rate: 18. On abdominal examination patient's abdominal contour was flat, on auscultation normal peristaltic sound can be heard in all 4 quadrant, on percussion there was normal resonating sound in bowel area and dull note over liver and spleen area, on palpation there was no hepatomegaly or splenomegaly noted. At this stage consulting doctor conducted Complete Blood Count analysis which showed high Eosinophils. Based on this stool sample for staining and following results were found.

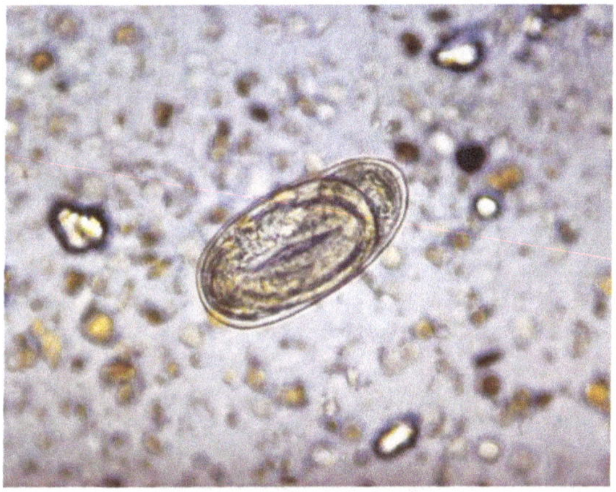

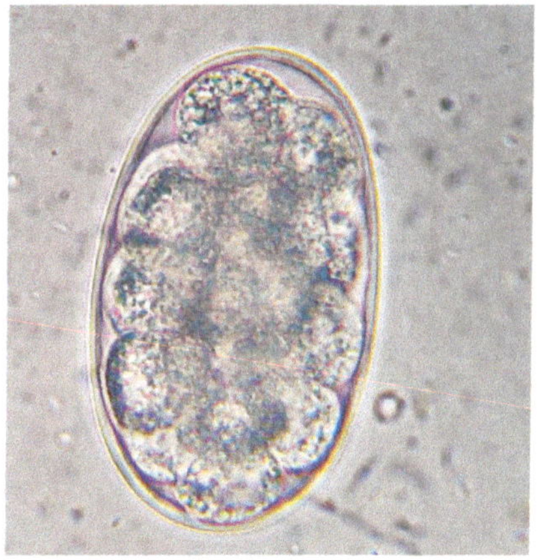

Source: Wikipedia; Author: Joel Mills

What is the drug of choice for this patient?

A. Sulphadiazine
B. Praziquantel
C. Acyclovir
D. Albendazole

Answer: D. Albendazole

Solution

- This is the case of infection caused by hookworm.
- Two classical species of hookworm are:
  1. Ancyclostoma duodenale.
  2. Necator americanus.
- **Habitat:** Jejunum.
- **Host:** Human.
- **Mode of infection:** Skin penetration.
- **Infective form:** Filariform larvae.

Clinical Presentation:

1. Abdominal pain.
2. Diarrhea.
3. Loeffler syndrome.

Diagnosis:

- Hookworm's egg with 4-8 blastomere in stool.
- **Drug of Choice:** Albendazole.

98. 22 years old male comes with primary complain of watery diarrhea for the last 7 days. There is no presence of abdominal pain. There is no history of associated nausea or vomiting neither there is any presence of pus or blood on stool. There is no history of recent travel. But he visited a restaurant 10 days ago to have beef and rice for dinner. Patient is non alcoholic, non smoker with no known history of drug abuse. Patient has been hypertensive for the last 10 years and have been on ACE inhibitor since then. On physical examination patient looks dull with no signs of dehydration. But his vitals are stable with Pulse rate of 78, Blood Pressure of 124/88, respiratory rate of 18 and his temperature was 99°C.

There is no presence of icterus in the eye neither there is presence of any other sign of jaundice. His Complete Blood Count analysis showed increased Eosinophils and stools examination shows following presentation.

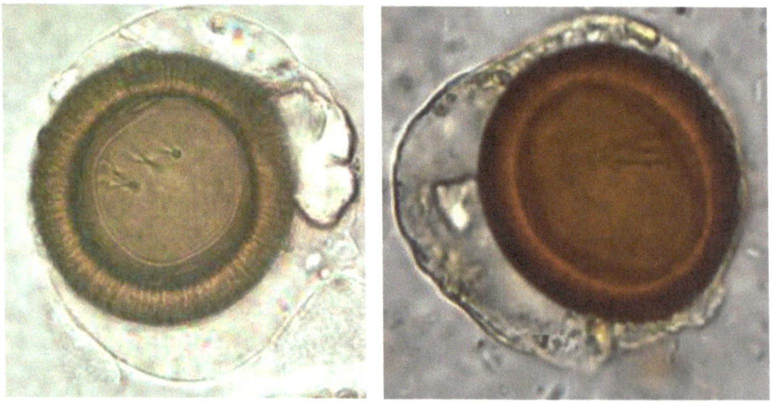

What is the infective form of pathogenic organism?

A. Cysticercus bovis
B. Rhabditiform larvae
C. Filariform larvae
D. Egg

Answer: A. Cysticercus bovis

Solution

- This is the case of infection caused by Taenia saginata.
- Taenia saginata comes under the classification of 'Cestodes'.
- **Definitive host:** Human's small intestine.
- **Infective form:** Cysticercus bovis.

Clinical Presentation:

1. Abdominal pain.
2. Diarrhea.
3. Anorexia.

Diagnosis:

- Stool test shows characteristic egg as shown below.

Treatment:

- Niclosamide, praziquantel.

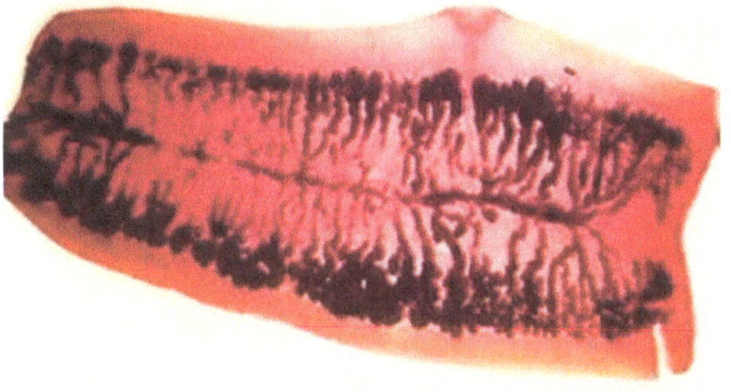

Mature proglottid of Taenia saginata

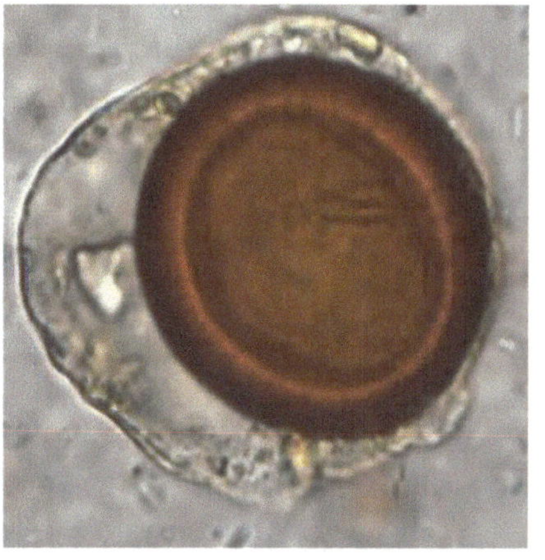

Taenia egg in Iodine stained wet mount in stool sample

99. 23 years old male comes with primary complain of headache for the last 3 days. Headache is throbbing in nature persisting in the occipital region. Headache was resistant to NSAIDs. He had suffered such headache before since childhood but he used to get relieved within 1-2 hours. There is no associated visual disturbance or loss of coordination or loss of perception. Neither there is any history of incontinence. Patient was born at tertiary care unit and his birth was uneventful via normal vaginal delivery. Patient vaccine status is complete. Between the age of 13 and 18 patient experienced 5-6 episodes and of sudden falling down while walking. Patient has stuck to his normal routine diet. Patient has no associated history of recent trauma. There is no history of recent travel neither he has consumed poorly cooked meat in recent times. On physical examination patient BMI was normal with stable vitals pulse rate of 75, Blood Pressure of 128/90, respiratory rate of 18. There is no peculiar lesion or rash found on patient. On ophthalmic examination there was no sign of papilledema. On neurological examination there was no presence of neck stiffness or Kernig's sign or Brudzinski sign neither was there any presence of café au lait spots.

As for the higher mental function assessment patient was oriented in time, place and person, he was having normal attention and calculation ability, his register and recall ability was intact. Patient was able to understand and follow the command. His speech and language was intact. All his Cranial Nerves were intact. As for his trunk and limb assessment, upon inspection there was no postural inability, wasting or hypertrophy was noted. Neither was there any presence of scar or movement abnormality found. His tone and power in limbs were intact. Patient had no abnormal reflexes.

As for his cerebellar abnormality there was no presence of dysdiadochokinesia or nystagmus or ataxia or dysmetria or hypotonia or past pointing test or rebound phenomenon or rhomberg test all these tests and assessment were found to be negative.

No other sensory abnormality was found. As for gait his gait was broadbased with his foot moving outward and stuck/rubbing the ground. He had a normal Glasgow Coma Score.

At this stage consulting doctor conducted NCCT of head which showed isodense structure in ventricles.

Now the consulting doctor conducted lumbar puncture which came out to be increased and CSF was positive for T. solium serology. Which of the following is wrong with regards to pathogenic organism?

A. Infective form is cysticercus cellulosae

B. Generally occur by having raw uncooked pork

C. Drug of Choice: Albendazole

D. Cause hydatid cyst

Answer: D. Cause hydatid cyst

Solution

- This is the case of Taenia solium infection causing Cysticercosis.
- **Mode of infection** of Taenia solium is ingestion of Cysticercus cellulosae present in poorly cooked pork or contaminated water.
- **Sites for Cysticercosis:** Muscle (Most common), brain and spinal cord.
- **Clinical presentation** can be very varied and depends on site of infection.
- In brain it can cause partial seizure, headache, visual symptoms etc.

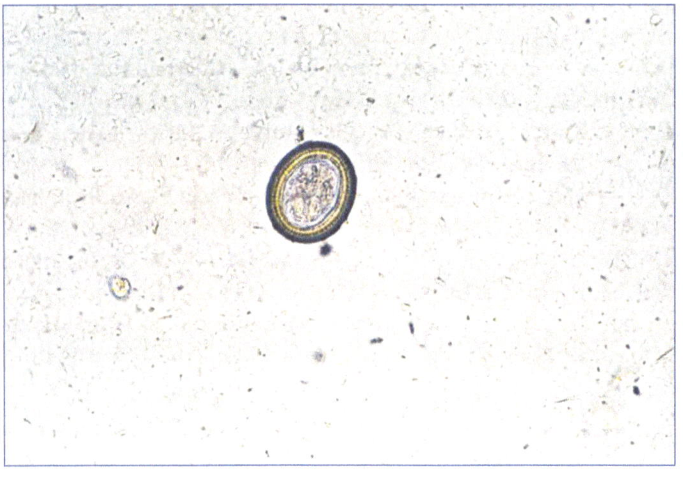

Taenia solium ovum

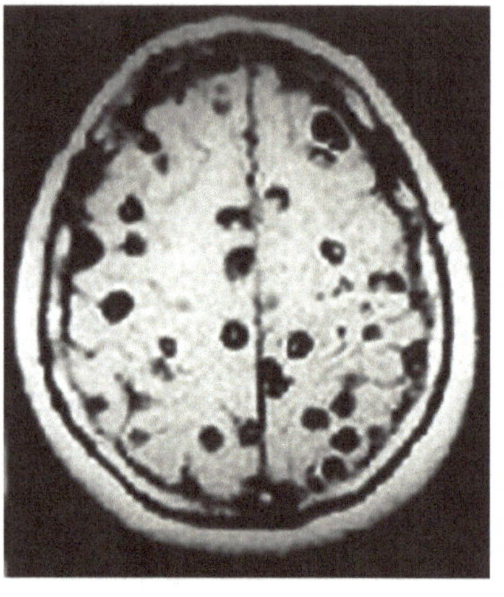

MRI showing Neurocysticercosis

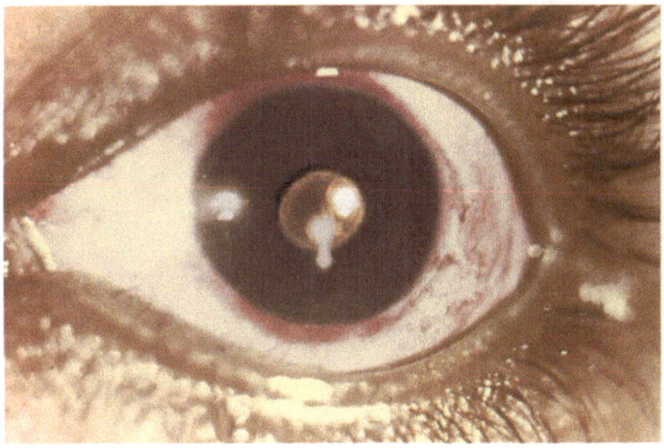

Larvae for Taenia solium in the pupil

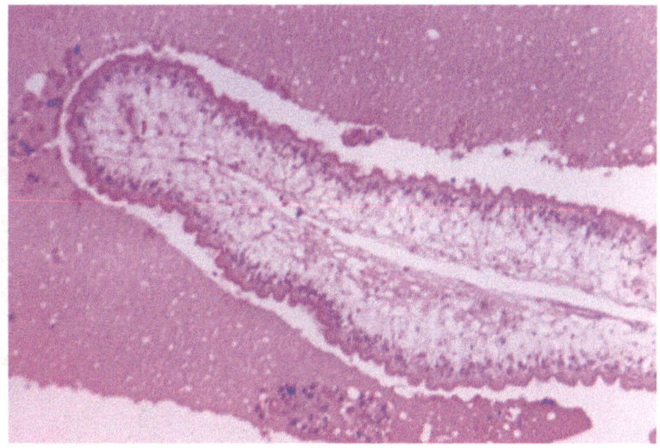

Brain biopsy of neurocysticercosis

Diagnosis:

- Stool sample showing presence of T. solium egg.
- CT and MRI showing Neurocysticercosis.

Treatment:

- Nicolazamide or Praziquantel for T. solium infection.
- Albendazole or Praziquantel for neurocysticercosis.

100. 32 years old female was admitted to hospital with primary complain of abdominal pain in right hypochondrial region along with nausea and vomiting for last 16 hours. Pain is continuous and sharp in nature. There is no associated diarrhea or abnormal bowel movement. There is no history of jaundice or hepatic disorder. On physical examination patient vitals were stable with Pulse rate of 73, Blood Pressure of 122/88, respiratory rate of 18 and normal temperature. There was no sign of icterus in the eye. On conducting Complete Blood Count analysis and LFT nothing abnormal was found. At this stage hepatic Ultrasound was done which showed presence of cyst with detached membrane or water Lilly sign or floating membrane sign. Which of the following is NOT correct regarding the pathogenic organism?

A. Definitive host for pathogenic organism is human

B. Pathogenic organism

C. First line management is PAIR

D. Accidental intermediate host are human

Answer: A. Definitive host for pathogenic organism is human

Solution

- This is the case of Hydatid cyst caused by Echinococcus granulosus.
- **Definitive host:** Dog.
- Man is the accidental intermediate host.
- **Organs affected:** Liver (most common) > lungs.
- **Symptoms and signs:**

1. Abdominal pain.
2. Nausea and vomiting.
3. Hepatomegaly.

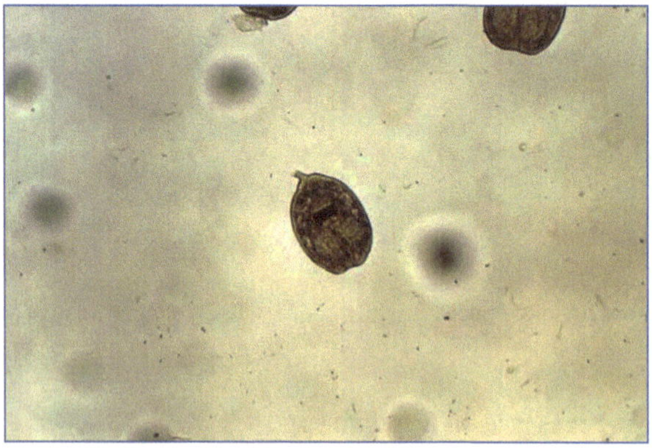

Image of Echinococcus liberated from hydatid cyst

Treatment:

- **Drug of Choice:** Albendazole.
- **Procedure of Choice:** PAIR (Percutaneous Aspiration Injection and Reaspiration).

101. 45 years old male comes with multiple complain of intermittent fever and malaise related symptoms along with progressive generalized weakness for the last 7 months. He has also been loosing weight for the last 2 months, in the last 2 months he has lost 15 kg. Patient is non alcoholic, non smoker with no known drug abuse. On physical examination patient looks dull. There was presence of generalised lymphadenopathy. There is no sign of icterus or any other sign of jaundice or hepatic disease. His vitals were pulse rate 90, Blood Pressure: 110/82, respiratory rate of 19/min. At this stage Complete Blood Count analysis was conducted which showed Pancytopenia, Hypergammaglobulinemia, no atypical cells were found. At this stage doctor decided to conduct Bone marrow biopsy which showed following image of Leishmania donovani body in cytoplasm of macrophage.

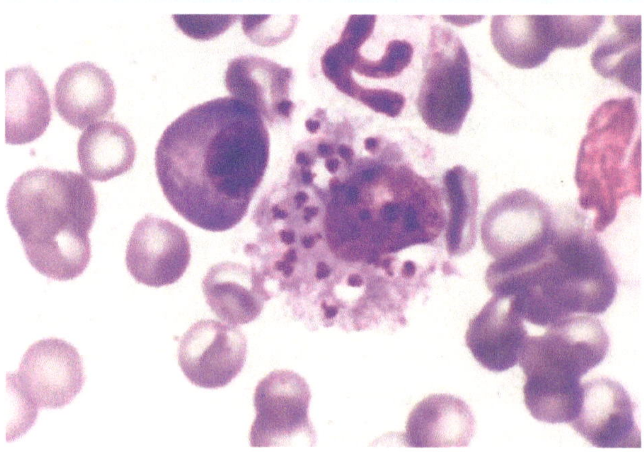

Which of the following is NOT correct regarding pathogenic organism?

A. Above mentioned condition is caused by Leishmania donovani complex (L. donovani, L.infantum, L. chagasi)

B. Vector is phlebotomus argentipes

C. Site of latency is B-cell

D. Albumin : Globulin ratio is reversed

E. Confirmatory diagnosis can be done by doing ELISA for recombinant antigen rK-39

Answer: C. Site of latency is B-cell

Solution

- This is the case of Visceral leishmania/Kala azar.
- **Definitive host:** Humans.
- **Habitat:** Reticuloendothelial cells.
- **Vector:** Sandfly.
- **Infective form:** Promastigote.
- **Mode of Transmission:** Bite of sandfly, blood transfusion, through placenta.

Pathophysiology:

- Promastigote gets phagocytosed by Reticuloendothelial cells/macrophages and gets converted into amastigotes which undergoes binary fission and eventually causing the cell to rupture.
- If no immune response/antibody present then it again gets phagocytosed by macrophage and undergoes repeated cycles.

Clinical Features:

- Incubation period is of 3-5 months:
    1. Persistent intermittent fever.
    2. Progressive weight loss.
    3. Malaise related symptoms.

Diagnosis:

- Complete Blood Count analysis shows Pancytopenia (It occurs because Bone marrow contains proliferating macrophage containing amastigotes).
- Hypergammaglobulinemia causing reversible albumin : globulin ratio.
- Best specimen to observe leishmania inside macrophage is not blood.
- To observe and diagnose Kala azar following specimen should be considered:
    - o Bone marrow > lymph node.
- Under giemsa stain or leishmania stain we will be able to observe 'Leishmania donovani body' inside of macrophage which is actually kinetoplast or mitochondrial DNA of Leishmania.
- **Cultivation:** Novy-MacNeal-Nicolle medium.
- **Molecular methods of diagnosis:** NAAT's, ELISA for rK39 antigen.

Treatment:

- **Drug of Choice:** Amphotericin B.
  - o Oral miltefosine.
  - o Antimony compound.
  - o Sitamaquine.

102. 55 years old male is brought to ER with complain of chest pain. The attending doctor performs an ECG which came out to be normal and sends the blood for troponin test.

On taking history patient told that chest pain was mild to moderate in nature that was followed by intense coughing.

He also gives history of cough, hemoptysis and dyspnea for the last 2 days.

Patient is chronic smoker and smokes 1 packet each for the last 30 years.

Patient is non alcoholic with no known drug abuse. Patient is diabetic for the last 20 years and have been on metformin for the last 20 years and glifozin for the last 7 years. Patient has recently recovered from COVID infection (along with double pneumonia) 2 weeks back, he remained on insulin for 10 days.

Based on the given history doctor conduct chest X-ray along with sputum smear for giemsa staining which gave following findings:

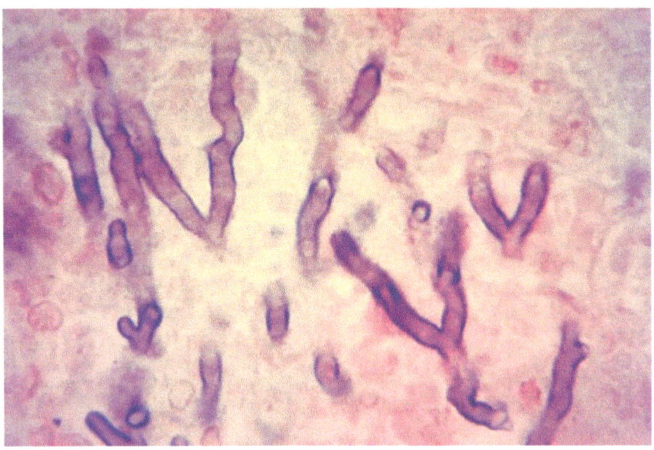

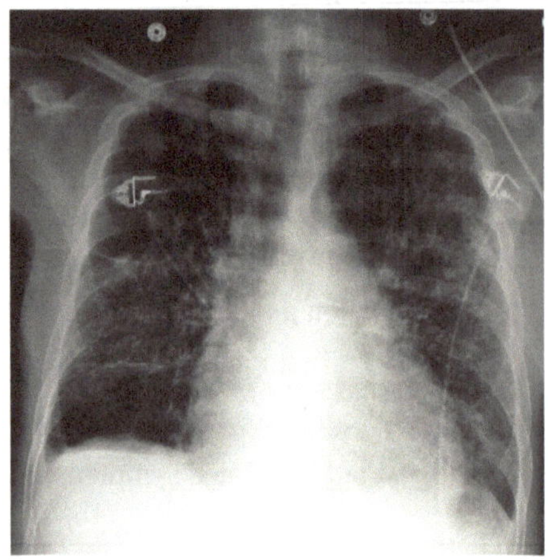

What should be the next step in management?

A. Start Voriconazole and then do confirmatory diagnosis

B. Perform confirmatory diagnosis then start Voriconazole

C. Start IV penicillin

Answer: A. Start Voriconazole and then do confirmatory diagnosis

Solution

- The given case is of invasive aspergillus.

- Aspergillus is ubiquitous infection which generally affects immunocompromised individuals.
- **Infective form:** Aspergillus conidia.
- On smear the most characteristic feature of aspergillus is hyaline septate mold along with dichotomous branching at acute angle.
- Although many species of aspergillus are pathogenic to human but there are 4 predominant species:

  1. Aspergillus Niger.
  2. Aspergillus flavus.
  3. Aspergillus fumigatus.
  4. Aspergillus terreus.
- The species that is Most Common Cause for invasive aspergillosis is Aspergillus fumigatus.
- **Diagnosis:** Giemsa staining.
- PCR for antigen detection Galactomannan.
- **ELISA:** Beta 1,3 D glycan.
- Cultivation media used for aspergillus is Sabouraud dextrose agar.
- **Drug of Choice:** Voriconazole.

103. 25 years old male comes to ENT department with complain of otalgia, irritation, itching in right ear for the last 7 days along with scanty discharge. Patient has recently started working in forest department. Patient has recovered from COVID 19 almost 15 days ago, he was given prednisolone for 7 days. Patient is non diabetic with no history of hypertension. On otoscopy it was noted that patient was having growth in External Auditory Canal, hyperemia of tympanic membrane along with small perforation. Consulting Doctor was suspicious of fungal infection and sends the discharge for giemsa staining which showed following findings:

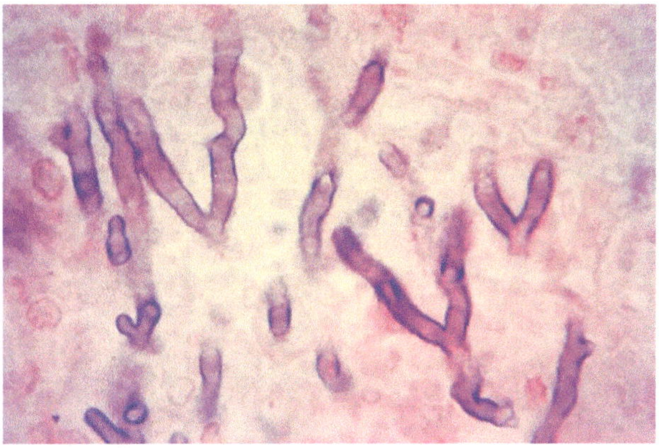

Based on this consulting doctor ask you what can be the most lethal complication that can occur in this patient due to this infection?

A. Perforation can lead to hearing loss

B. It can progress to invasive aspergillosis in immunocompromised patients which can even be life threatening

C. Can grow into massive lump and further decrease hearing ability of patient

Answer: B. It can progress to invasive aspergillosis in immunocompromised patients which can be life threatening

Solution

- The given case is that of otomycosis caused by aspergillus.
- Most common species of aspergillus causing otomycosis is Aspergillus Niger.
- One of the most pathognomic feature of otomycosis that help to differentiate from bacterial ear infection is otalgia and intense itchy.
- Aspergillus otomycosis generally occurs in individual living in places of high humidity and in malnourished children.
- **Treatment:** Topical Voriconazole.

104. 35 years old female was hospitalized due to pneumonia associated covid, during the morning rounds patient complains of headache, nasal congestion and visual impairment.

Patient was on steroid therapy. Patient is diabetic for the last 12 years and is on 3 times insulin in a day along with metformin and dapaglifozin. On examination one sided facial swelling was noticed, there was no proptosis, no cranial nerve palsy. Patient referred for MRI which showed soft tissue thickness along paranasal sinus along with gas fluid levels. What would be Drug of Choice in this case?

A. Liposomal amphotericin
B. Voriconazole
C. Amphotericin B
D. Praziquantel

Answer: C. Amphotericin B

105. 25 years old female comes to gynae department with complain of vaginal itching or soreness, abnormal vaginal discharge for the last 3 days. Patient is not married and never had any sexual intercourse. She has a family history of breast cancer for which she has been on OCP. Since this is the case of non STD type of genital infection, therefore doctor were highly suspicious for candida vaginal infection. Consulting doctor sends discharge specimen for staining and other 'test' which came out to be positive image given below.

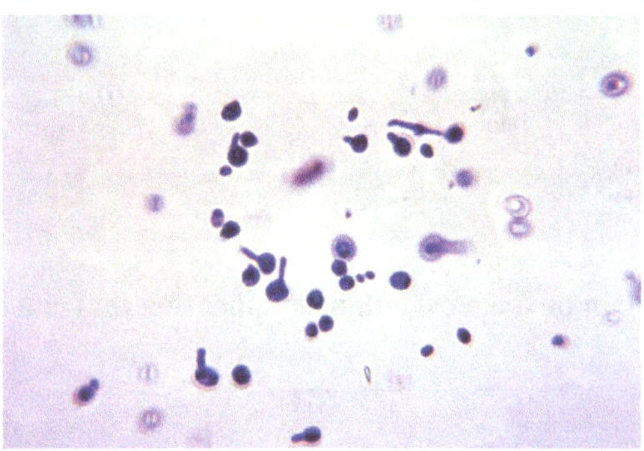
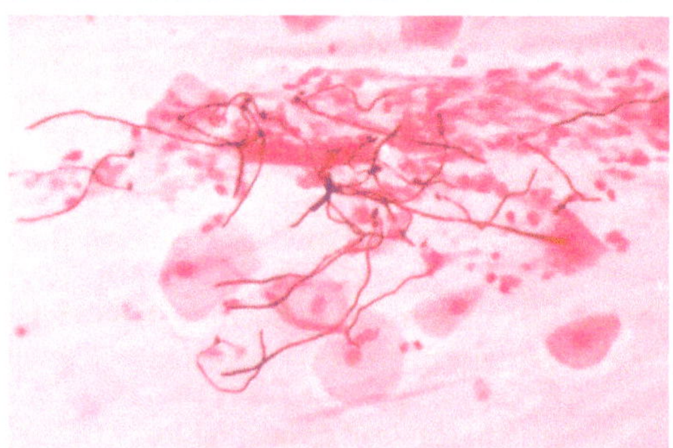

Name the test shown in image and stain used for pathogenic organism.

A. Nagler's reaction
B. McFadyean's reaction
C. Dinger's reaction
D. Germ tube test or Reynold Braude's reaction

Answer: D. Germ tube test or Reynold Braude's reaction

Solution

- The given case is that of genital infection caused by vaginal candidiasis.
- Candida is found as a normal flora of female genital tract, GIT, skin and oral cavity. It becomes pathogenic only when there is decrease in immunity of the patient, change in the hormonal status of female which can occur by pregnancy or use of OCP.
- Vaginal candidiasis is generally not associated with sexual transmission.
- Candida morphologically is yeast like fungi.
- For cultivation of candida Sabaraud dextrose agar is used which gives 'Off white pasty' colonies.
- There are many types of candida species.
- Few of the most important candida species in terms of human pathogenicity:
    - o Candida albicans.
    - o Candida dubliniensis.
    - o Candida krusei.
    - o Candida auris.
- Candida albicans and Candida dubliniensis can be differentiated by Germ tube test or Reynold Braude's phenomenon.
- To further differentiate Candida albicans and Candida dubliniensis we utilise the property of candida albicans to grow at 45°C and to grow in hypertonic saline.
- We can also use CHROM agar to differentiate each species of candida.
- Each species give different colour on chrom agar.
- **Treatment:** Azoles.

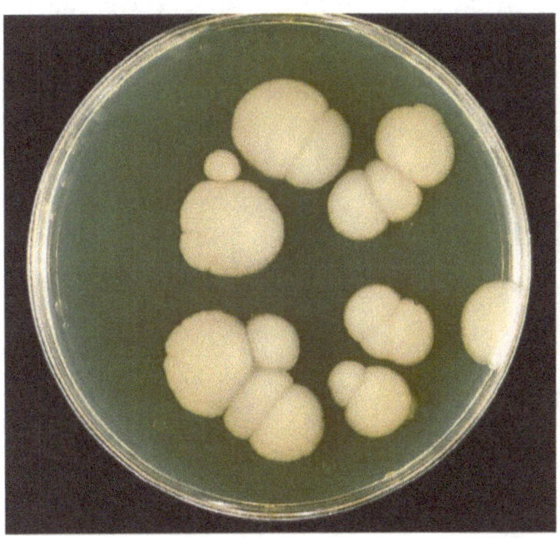

SABHI agar plate culture

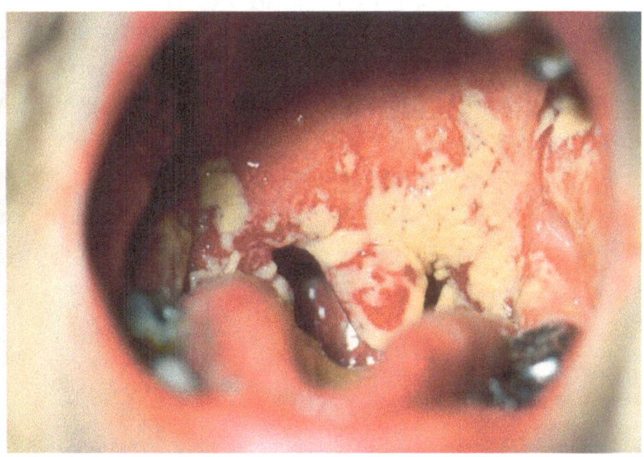

Oral thrush caused by Candida albicans infection

106. 33 years old male comes with complain of altered mental status, neck stiffness, increase irritability and headache for the last 2 days. Patient denies any head trauma. Patient has recently recovered from COVID 1 week back, he remained on steroids (prednisolone) for 5 days. Patient denies being infected by any other infection in recent past. Patient is non smoker, non alcoholic with no known drug abuse. Patient is non diabetic with no complain of hypertension. On physical examination his vitals were stable but a lesion was seen on his labium. Based on this your senior doctor asks you what is the site of latency of the causative organism?

A. Sacral ganglion
B. Lymphocytes
C. Secretory glands
D. Trigeminal ganglion

Answer: D. Trigeminal ganglion

Solution

- The given case is that of reactivation of HSV - 1 infection due to steroids given to curb hyperimmune response initiated by COVID.
- Herpes simplex virus 1 like all HSV is an ubiquitous infection.
- **Mode of Infection** for HSV-1 is oropharyngeal route.
- Latency for HSV-1 occurs in Trigeminal ganglion.
- **Clinical presentation** of primary infection of HSV-1 includes gingivostomatitis and pharyngitis. Also there can be vesicle formation.
- **Clinical presentation** of reactivation of HSV 1 infection manifest as herpes labialis.
- Severe cases of HSV can also cause encephalitis (as shown in this case).
- **Diagnosis:** Can be made by immunofluorescence or in case of lesion or vesicles we can take scrapings of lesion or vesicle and check for presence of Tzank cell (multi-nucleated giant cells) on staining.
- If there is CNS involvement then we can do CSF NAAT.
- **Treatment:** Acyclovir or valacyclovir.

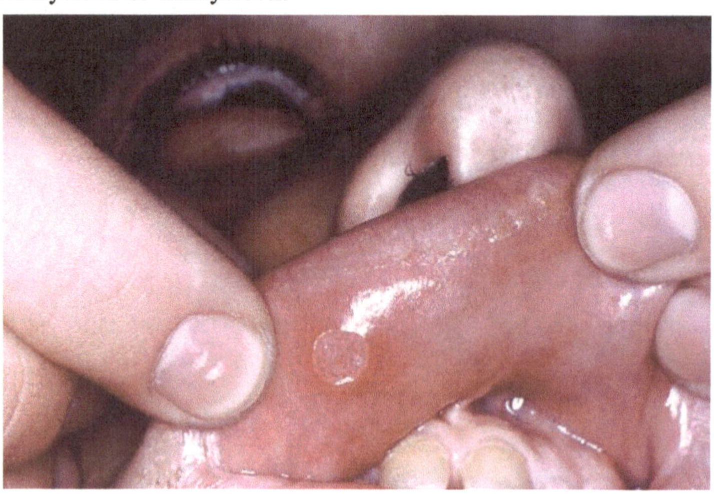

Herpes affecting oral cavity

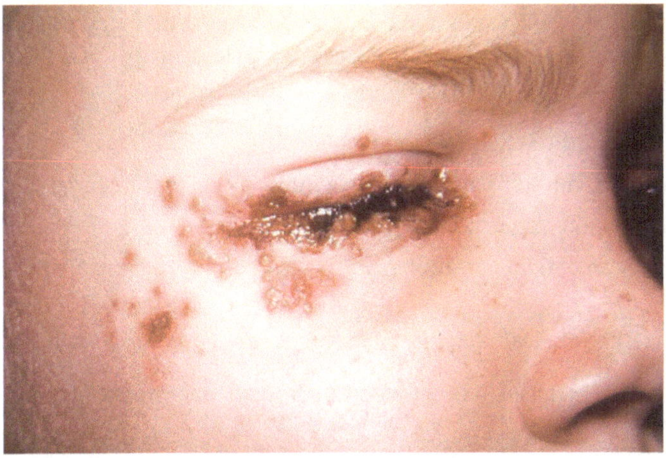

Herpes affecting face and eye

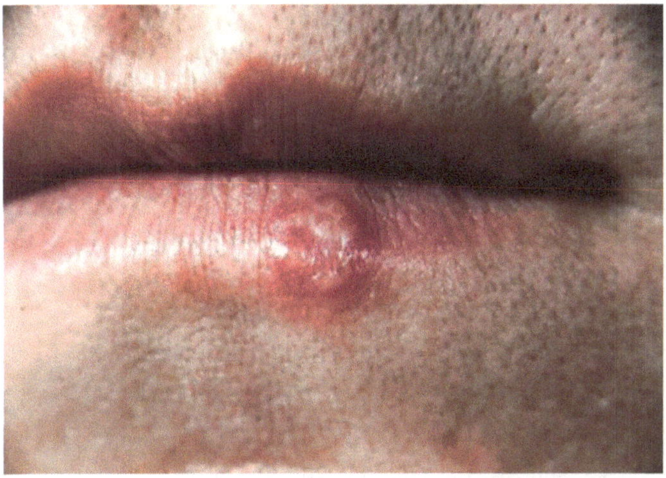

Herpes labialis

107. 6 years old child is brought to OPD with rashes on both cheeks and reticular rashes on upper limb as shown in image.

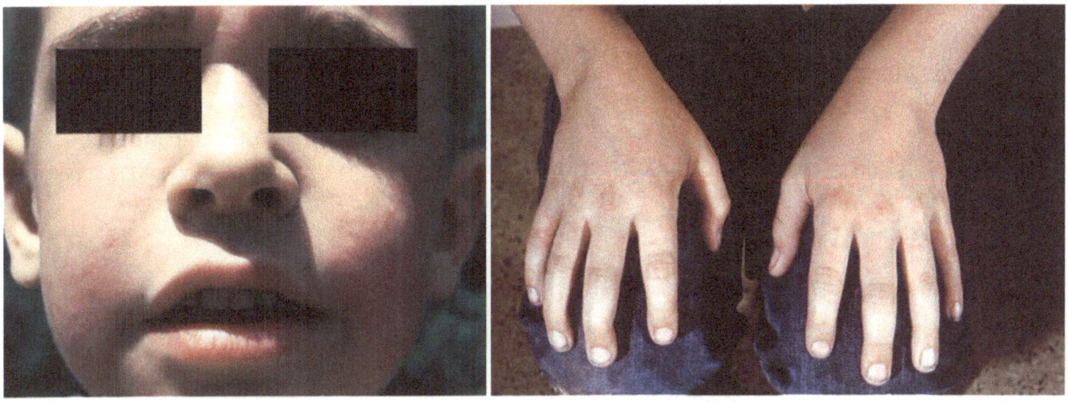

Child was born via normal vaginal delivery at 37 weeks; delivery was uneventful and child's vaccine status is also complete. At this stage your professor ask you which of the following is NOT correct regarding pathogenic organism?

A. Receptor for parvovirus is 'P' group antigen

B. Primary infection in children cause Erythema infectiosum or fifth disease

C. No intervention required spontaneous resolution seen in 5-7 days

D. Primary infection in children or adolescent is also known to cause 'Papular purpuric gloves and sick syndrome'

E. Aplastic anemia like clinical scenario can never occur due to parvovirus infection

Answer: E. Aplastic anemia like clinical scenario can never occur due to parvovirus infection

Solution

- This is the case of 'fifth disease' or 'erythema infectiosum' caused by parvovirus.
- Parvovirus is ubiquitous infection.
- **Mode of Transmission:** Respiratory.
- As for the clinical presentation is concerned parvovirus can cause different types of pathology like:
  1. In childhood it causes Erythema infectiosum which manifest as fever, malaise, slapped cheek rash along with reticular rash on limbs (as shown in image).
     - **Diagnosis** by serology.
     - Spontaneous resolution seen within 1 week.
  2. In children or adolescent it causes 'papular purpuric gloves socks syndrome'.
     - Here we see painful pruritic symmetrical swelling on hands and feet (as shown in image).
     - **Diagnosis:** Serology.
  3. In adults we see symmetrical small joint arthropathies.
     - **Most common:** Wrist and fingers.
     - **Diagnosis:** Serology.

108. 40 years old female present with complain of fever and malaise related symptoms. Patient received renal transplant 1 month back due to CKD which was caused by uncontrolled Diabetic mellitus. Patient is currently on immunosuppressant regime of Tacrolimus and prednisolone. Patient vitals were stable with slightly increased pulse rate of 91, Blood Pressure of 145/88 and respiratory rate being 14/min. On physical examination patient is oriented in time, place and person but looked pale, there was no sign of icterus. Based on this consulting doctor send blood for Complete Blood Count which revealed increased reticulocytes, decrease haptoglobin, increase in LDH-1, neutrophils 30%, lymphocytes 50%. What is most probable cause for patient's condition?

A. Parvovirus infection causing pure red cell aplasia

B. Autoimmune hemolysis

C. Drug induced anemia

D. Hemolytic Uremic Syndrome

Answer: A. Parvovirus infection causing pure red cell aplasia

Solution

- This is the case of Pure Red Cell Aplasia.
- This is seen in case of parvovirus causing primary infection in immunocompromised individual getting attached to 'P' blood group antigen causing hemolysis and fall in Hemoglobin.
- **Diagnosis:** Polymerase Chain Reaction.
- **Treatment:** Immunoglobulins.

109. At 27 weeks of pregnancy pregnant female underwent fetal ultrasound which showed severe anemia along with thickened placenta and large amniotic fluid. Mother denies any sort of small joint arthropathy. She also denied any sort of family history related to inherited blood disorder. At this stage doctor conducts mother's Complete Blood Count analysis which showed neutrophils 30% and lymphocytes 60% and send for parvovirus serology which came out to be positive. Which of the following is correct regarding parvovirus?

A. It causes papular purpuric gloves and sock syndrome

B. It can cause chorioretinitis in infant which would have pizza pie retinopathy or cottage cheese and sauce appearance

C. It can cause cicatrizing or scaring skin lesion

D. Receptor for parvovirus is CD-155

Answer: A. It causes papular purpuric gloves and sock syndrome

Solution

- This is the case of parvovirus infecting pregnant mother in first half of pregnancy and causing transplacental transmission that eventually lead to fetal hydrops.
- Parvovirus gets attached to RBC via 'P' blood group antigen.

110. 70 years old male came to Emergency room saying that he wake up in morning with weakness on right side of face along with drooping eyebrows and mouth, drooling on affected side, inability to close eyelid on affected side and absent forehead wrinkles on affected side. Patient gives a history that last night he had right sided headache with pain extending to right ear for which he took NSAIDs and went to sleep. There is no history of loss of vision or double vision, there is no history of recently 1 month back patient has been diagnosed with CML for which he is on chemotherapy regime of hydroxyurea. There is no other sign or symptoms of autoimmune condition present in personal or family history. Patient is non smoker, non alcoholic drinker with no known history of drug abuse. On clinical examination vitals were within normal range with pulse of 72, blood pressure of 120/85. There were no remarkable findings on CNS examination. Based on this the attending doctor wanted to rule out any possibility of stroke and Multiple Sclerosis so doctor conducted CT and MRI of brain which showed no sign of Multiple Sclerosis or stroke. Consulting doctor was highly suspecious for reactivation of zoster varicella virus. What special type of shingles is patient suffering with?

A. Herpes zoster ophthalmicus
B. Ramsay Hunt syndrome
C. Zoster sine herpete
D. Herpes encephalitis

Answer: B. Ramsay Hunt syndrome

Solution

- The given case is of special type of zoster called Ramsay Hunt syndrome.
- Generally occurs due to reactivation of zoster of geniculate ganglion.
- **Characteristic Feature:** Bell's palsy, vesicles in External Auditory Canal and tympanic membrane, can also cause hearing loss, vitiligo, otalgia and loss of taste in anterior ⅔rd of tongue.
- **Treatment:** Acyclovir, prednisolone.

Other Options:

- Herpes zoster ophthalmicus–>special type of zoster that involve ophthalmic branch of Trigeminal nerve.
- Zoster sine herpete–> special type of zoster where there is no lesion but pain present.

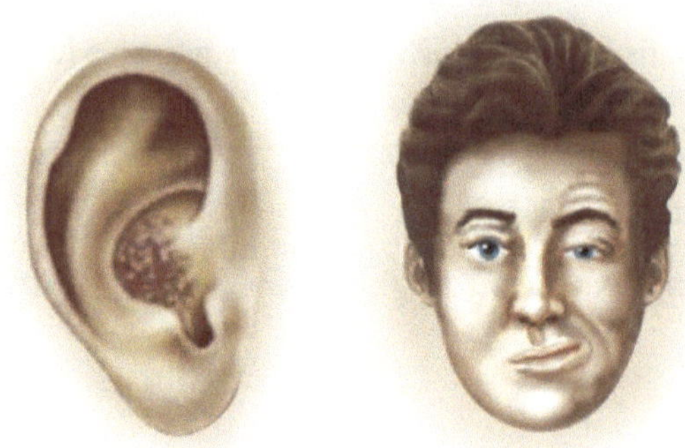

Ramsay Hunt syndrome

Source: http://openi.nlm.nih.gov/detailedresult.php?img=3847606_1756-0500-6-337-2&query=ramsay%20 hunt&it=xg&lic=by&req=4&npos=3, Author: Worme M, Chada R, Lavallee L, Creative Commons Attribution: 2.0 Generic license

111. Gravida 2 Para 2 female gave birth to a child 2 days ago in a tertiary care unit in rural areas of state of Bihar, India via normal vaginal delivery. Now she present with multiple complain of sudden generalised vesicular eruption along with altered mental status and confusion, neck rigidity and dyspnea since early morning. Neonate also developed high fever and vesicular lesion with surrounding erythema which looked like dew drop on rose petal appearance. These lesions were dominant on trunk and flexors. Based on these doctor sends scrapings of base of vesicular lesion for giemsa staining which showed multiple nucleated giant cell, i.e., Tzanck smear. At this stage your professor ask you what is the Treatment of Choice for this patient and which prophylactic vaccine should have been given to the patient?

A. Acyclovir; Zostavax
B. Immunoglobulins; Varivax
C. Acyclovir; Varivax
D. Immunoglobulins; Zostavax

Answer: D. Immunoglobulins; Zostavax

Solution

- This is the case of Perinatal/neonatal varicella syndrome.
- This is seen when mother develops varicella 7 days before and 2 days after delivery.
- **Clinical Presentation:**
    1. Disseminated Disease (In the given case patient have dyspnea which can be due to pneumonia).
    2. Generalised vesicular eruption.
    3. Child will also develop vesicular eruption along with high fever.
- **Diagnosis:** Giemsa staining of scrapings of base of vesicular lesion showing Tzanck smear.
- **Treatment:** Immunoglobulins.
- Prophylaxis that should have been given to female would be Varivax vaccine.

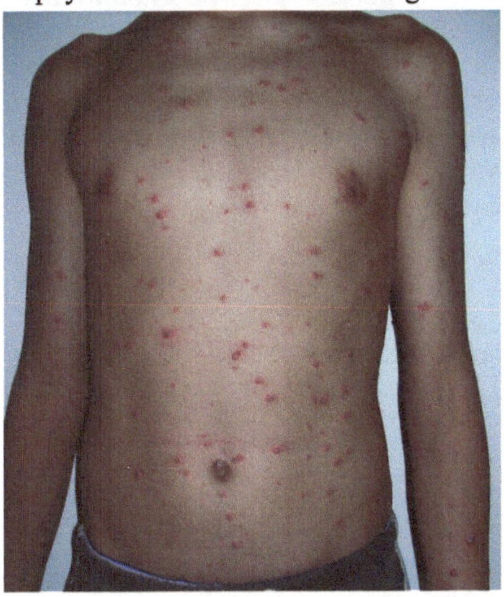

Varicella

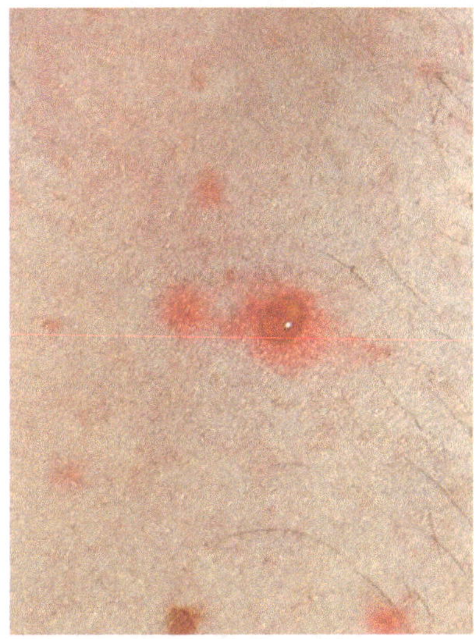

Dew on rose petal appearance

Source: Wikipedia; Author: F Malan, Creative Commons Attribution: ShareAlike 3.0 Unported license

112. 19 years old Gravida 2 para 1 at 15 weeks of gestation developed peculiar crop like eruption of vesicle surrounded by erythema that looked like dew drops on rose petal. Patient was started on Acyclovir. At this stage your professor ask you what are the complication that are possible in the offspring? (Multiple options can be correct).

A. Chorioretinitis
B. Hypoplastic limbs
C. Cerebral atrophy
D. Cicatrizing/scaring skin lesion
E. Omphalocele

Answer: A,B,C,D

Solution

- This is the case of fatal varicella syndrome or congenital varicella syndrome.

- Fatal Varicella Syndrome or Congenital Varicella Syndrome generally occurs when mother develops Varicella infection within first 20 weeks of gestation leading to certain defects in newborn like:
  1. Cerebral atrophy.
  2. Chorioretinitis.
  3. Hypoplastic limbs.
  4. Low birth weight.
  5. Cicatrizing or scaring skin lesion.

113. 37 years old male presents to OPD with multiple complains of fever and malaise related symptoms for last 7 days along with neck rigidity, photophobia and headache the for the last 2 days.There is no associated visual anomaly. Patient has a 20 days travel history to Japan where he got involved in various activities like camping in rural side skydiving etc. He does give history of multiple mosquito bite during his visit. Patient is non smoker, alcoholic consume 1 can of beer every day, with no history of drug abuse. Patient's vital were stable with Pulse rate 73, Blood Pressure of 138/88, respiratory rate of 22. On physical examination patient is oriented in time, place and person. No rash or lesion was spotted. Based on this doctor conducts Complete Blood Count analysis along with lumbar puncture which showed neutrophils 22% and lymphocytes 55% in blood. While CSF was clear, Glucose was more than ⅔rd of plasma glucose level and protein was minimally increased. At this stage consulting doctor send serology for EBV, mumps, measles, coxsackie, Enterovirus and Japanese Encephalitis Virus. Out of these IgM for Japanese Encephalitis Virus came out to be positive.

At this stage your professor ask you which of the following is NOT correct regarding this pathogenic organism?

A. Travelers are advised to be vaccinated before traveling to endemic areas

B. Vector-culex tritaeniorhynchus

C. Amplifying reservoir is pig

D. Ardeid (water) bird

E. Confirmatory diagnosis by blood culture

Answer: E. Confirmatory diagnosis by blood culture

Solution

- This is the case of Japanese Encephalitis Virus.
- **Epidemiology:** It is epidemic in East Asia.
- **Vector:** Culex tritaeniorhynchus.
- **Reservoir:** Ardeid birds.
- **Amplifying reservoir:** Pigs.

Clinical Presentation:

- **Incubation period:** 5-15 days.
- **Symptoms:** Malaise related symptoms, fever, nausea, vomiting etc.
- Later there is neurological manifestation like: Meningitis, Cranial Nerve palsy, speech abnormality, Parkinson like presentation and seizure.
- Mortality is 30%.
- Neurological sequelae in 50%.
- **Diagnosis:** Serology.

- **Confirmatory diagnosis:** PRNT (Plaque Reduction Neutralization Test).
- **Treatment** is symptomatic.
- Japanese Encephalitis Virus is part of Flavivirus.
- **Other Flaviviruses are:** West Nile Virus, St. Louis encephalitis.

114. 15 years old male was admitted with primary complain of fever, nausea vomiting and malaise related symptoms for the last 2 days along with neck stiffness and photophobia for the last few hours. Patient has a recent travel history to Australia where she was involved in activities like swimming, camping etc. He has returned from Australia 6 days ago. Patient is non smoker non alcoholic with no known history of drug abuse. On physical examination patient was confused and his vitals were pulse rate 88, blood pressure 122/88, respiratory rate 20. On conducting his neurological examination Kernig's sign and Brudzinski sign was positive, there was no presence of café au lait spots. As for his higher mental function assessment he was confused oriented in person but not in time and place. He was able to understand and follow the command. His language and speech was intact. All his Cranial Nerves were intact. His normal attention and calculation ability along with his register and recall ability was affected. On conducting his trunk and limb neurological assessment it was inspected that patient was having no muscle hypertrophy or wasting, there was abnormal scar or movement. His tone and power in limbs was normal and all his reflexes were intact.

On conducting his cerebellar examination there was no dysdiadochokinesia, no dysmetria or past pointing test was negative. No sign of nystagmus or ataxia. Rebound phenomenon test was negative. There were no sensory abnormality and gait was normal along with negative Romberg test. His GCS score was 11.

Based on this Complete Blood Count analysis and lumbar puncture was conducted. Nothing significant was found in Complete Blood Count but for lumbar puncture pressure was high and CSF was yellow turbid in color. Glucose was minimally increased (less than half of plasma glucose) and CSF protein was increased. Neutrophils were elevated while his lymphocytes levels were low.

At this stage diagnosis of bacterial meningitis was made. Patient was started on Penicillin, Ampicillin and ceftriaxone. Doctor send a serology test for streptococcus, listeria monocytogenes, Neisseria meningitis. All of them came out to be negative, also patient condition kept on deteriorating despite of antibiotics and his GCS eventually fell to 7. Later vancomycin was also added which proved not to be very helpful and patient condition kept on deteriorating eventually leading to death. Upon conducting autopsy following findings were made:

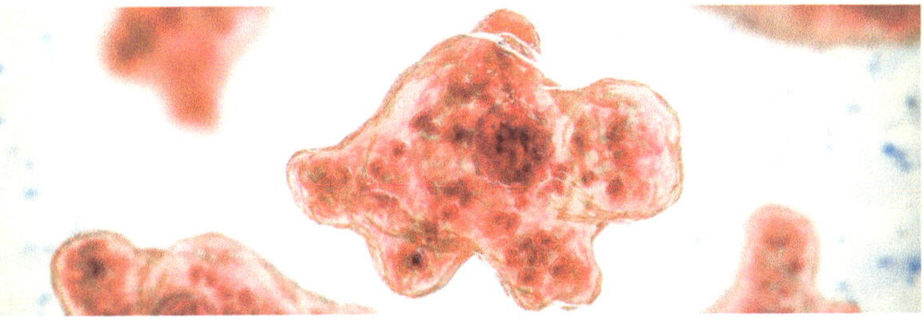

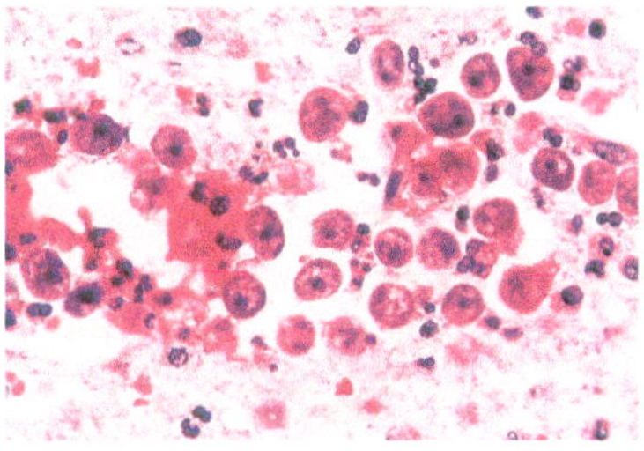

Based on this which of the following is NOT correct regarding pathogenic organism?

A. It can cause disease in immunocompetent patient

B. It mimics bacterial meningitis

C. Drug of choice: Amphotericin B + Rifampicin, azoles or miltefosine

D. It is non acid fast diplococci and have kidney shaped appearance

Answer: D. It is non acid fast diplococci and have kidney shaped appearance

Solution

- This is the case of Primary Amebic Meningoencephalitis that is caused by Naegleria fowleri also known as brain eating amoeba or amoeboflagellate.
- **Habitat:** Lakes or water body specially hot springs or where there thermal plant warm water discharge.
- **Infective form:** Trophozoites.
- **Mode of Infection:** Swimming in infected water causing Naegleria fowleri trophozites to enter through nose travelling via olfactory nerve to meninges.

Clinical Presentation:

1. Altered mental status.
2. Fever and malaise related symptoms.
3. Stiffness of neck.
4. Photophobia.
5. Higher mental function disorder.
6. Altered taste and smell.
7. Personality change.

Diagnosis:

- CSF microscopy shows ameboid trophozoites.
- Molecular methods like PCR.

Treatment:

- Amphotericin B + Rifampicin, azoles or miltefosine.
- Mortality is 40-60% hence in every deteriorating case of bacterial meningitis have high suspicion for Naegleria fowleri. Specially if there is associated history of swimming in natural water body.

115. 25 years old male comes with multiple complain of diarrhea along with mucous and small amount of blood, fever and abdominal pain in right hypochondrium for the last 7 days. He has increased bowel movement 2-3 times a day with mucous and few drops of blood. His fever has ranged between 100 and 101°C and his right hypochondrial abdominal pain is sharp radiating towards right shoulder. Patient is non alcoholic, non smoker with no history of drug abuse. 10 days ago patient travel to countryside to visit his family. During the visit he denies any mite or fly bite.

He has stuck to his normal dietary pattern. Patient is non diabetic and normotensive. Patient has no history of jaundice or any other hepatic pathology. On physical examination his face looks dull and ill, his vitals were stable with mild fever of 100.2°C, pulse rate of 78, blood pressure of 138/88, respiratory rate of 18, there is no sign of icterus or any other sign of jaundice. Based on this Complete Blood Count analysis was conducted which showed elevated levels of Eosinophils. Stool examination showed the following presentation:

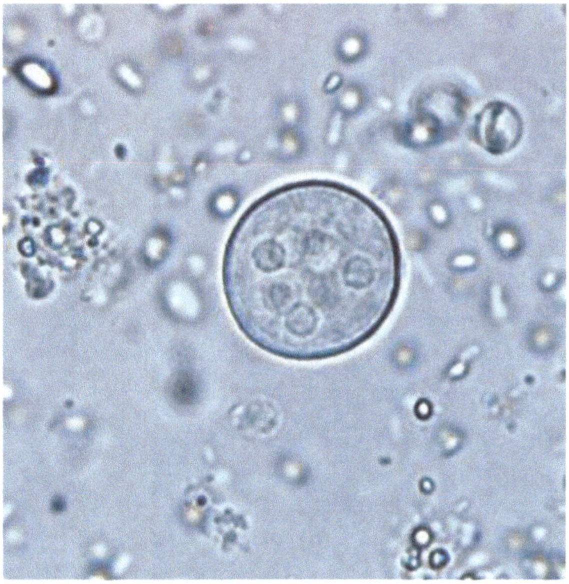

Hepatic CT shows following findings:

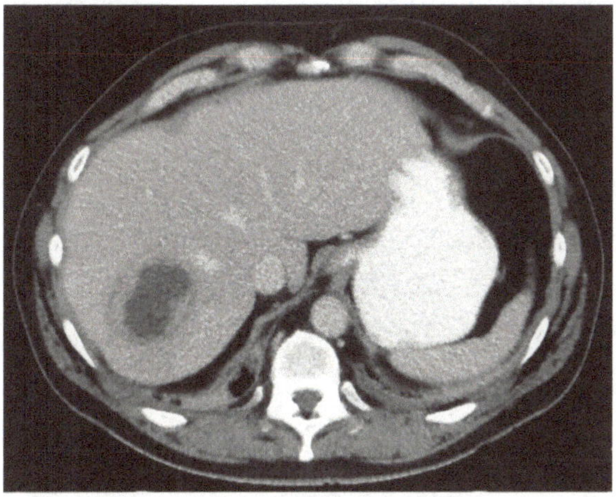

Doctor sends serology for EHEC, shigella, EIEC, Cryptosporidium, cyclospora and Entamoeba histolytica; out of which IgM for entamoeba histolytica came out to be positive.

Which of the following is NOT correct regarding pathogenic organism?

A. It is known to cause travelers' diarrhea

B. Infective form quadrinucleate cyst

C. Drug of choice: Metronidazole + paromomycin

D. Gharbi classification can be used for classifying amoebic liver abscess

E. Produce flask shaped or undermined ulcer

Answer: D. Gharbi classification can be used for classifying amoebic liver abscess

Solution

- This is the case of entamoeba histolytica of infection.
- Entamoeba histolytica is known to cause travelers' diarrhea and in some patients (around 5-10%) entamoeba histolytica can take a portal route and cause amoebic liver abscess.
- General characteristics of Entamoeba histolytica are:
  - o **Habitat:** Human's caecum or ascending colon.
  - o **Mode of Infection:** Feco-oral route.
  - o **Infective form:** Quadrinucleate cyst.
- Entamoeba histolytica also survives normal chlorination of water.
- Morphological appearance of Entamoeba histolytica:
  1. Eccentric nucleus along with central nucleolus.
  2. Fine chromatin spoke like linin.
  3. Food vacuole causing erythrophagocystosis.
- **Clinical Presentation:**
  1. Can be asymptomatic.
  2. Can cause Amoebic dysentery (diarrhea with blood and mucus).
  3. In few patients it can also cause amoebic liver abscess.
- Amoebic liver abscess is most common at posterosuperior surface of right hepatic lobe.

Diagnosis:

- Stool examination on saline and iodine mount showing presence of trophozoites and cysts.
- ELISA can be conducted for Gal/GalNAc lectin antigen.

Treatment:

- **Drug of Choice:** Metronidazole + Paromomycin/diloxanide furate (luminal amoebicide).

116. Patient come with following presentation:

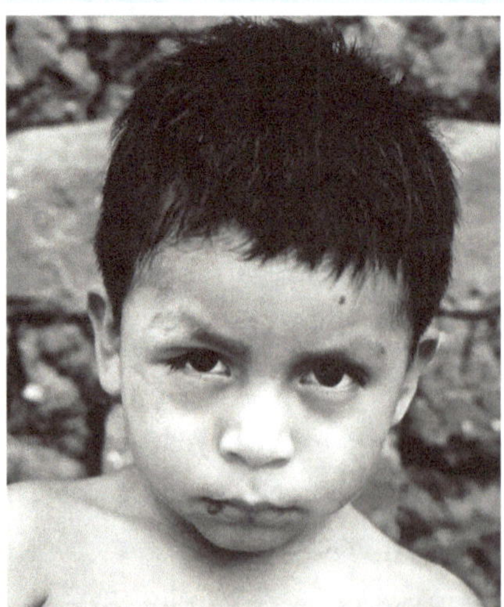

Patient also had fever along with malaise related symptoms for the last 2 days. Swelling around the eye is tender and her temperature was 101°C. She has a recent travel history to South America and has returned 15 days ago. During her holiday she was involved in multiple activities like camping in woods, mountaineering etc. Patient is non smoker non alcoholic with no history of known drug abuse. Which of the following statement is wrong with respect to patient's pathology?

A. Vector: Reduviid bug

B. Infective form: Metacyclic trypomastigote

C. Cause Romana's sign and chagoma

D. Chronic disease cause constrictive cardiomyopathy

Answer: D. Chronic disease cause constrictive cardiomyopathy

Solution

- This is the case of Chagas disease also known as South American trypanosomiasis trypanosoma cruzi.
- **Vector:** Reduviid.
- **Mode of Infection:** Percutaneous exposure to feces of bug.
- **Infective form:** Metacyclic trypomastigote.
- **Chagas disease (South American Trypanosomiasis): Incubation period:** 7-10 days.

Clinical Presentation:

- Painless erythematous swelling also known as chagoma.
- **Romana's sign:** Facial and eyelid swelling with ipsilateral lymphadenopathy.
- There can also be fever, malaise, anorexia with generalised lymphadenopathy.
- Myocarditis and hepatosplenomegaly may or may not be present.
- Acute Chagas can later lead on to chronic Chagas disease.
- Chronic Chagas can manifest as complication like dilated cardiomyopathy (most common), megacolon etc.

Diagnosis:

- Giemsa staining of blood shows trypomastigote.
- Other methods can be used like NAAT, immunofluorescence.
- For chronic Chagas we check for presence of IgG in serology via ELISA.

Treatment:

- **For acute case:** Nifurtimox or Benznidazole.
- **For chronic cases:** Treatment is symptomatic.

117. 35 years old male comes with primary complain of typical lesion as shown in image for last 20 days. Lesion was painless erythematous raised papule covered with crust and central ulcer. These lesions were present on face, hand and feet. There is no fever or any other associated

symptoms. Patient denied any mosquito bite neither there is any associated travel history. Patient denied getting in contact with any other patient with cutaneous pathology. Patient is non smoker, non alcoholic with no known history of drug abuse. On physical examination patient vitals were stable with Pulse rate of 73, Blood Pressure of 125/85, respiratory rate of 18. Based on this consulting doctor conducted biopsy for lesion which showed following findings:

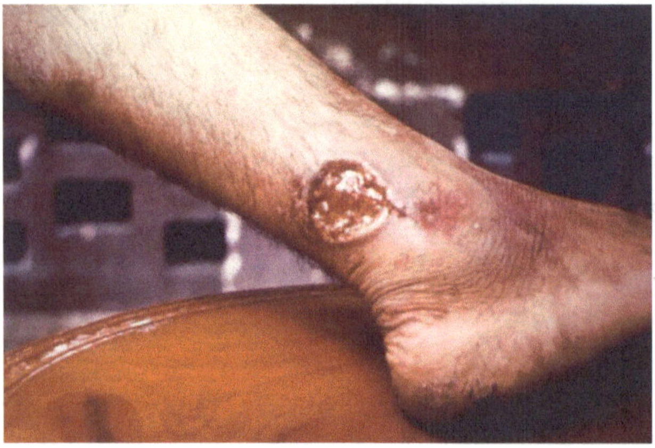

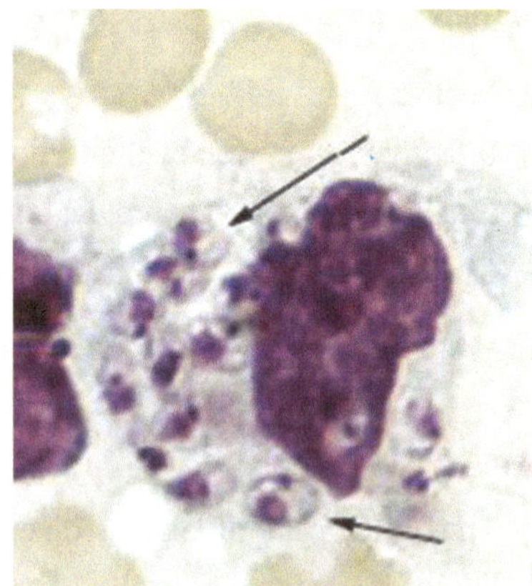

What is the pathological organism?

A. Leishmania tropica

B. Leishmania donovani

C. Trypanosoma cruzi

D. Coxsackie virus

Answer: A. Leishmania tropica

Solution

- This is the case of cutaneous Leishmania which is caused by Leishmania tropica complex that includes L. tropica, L. major, L. mexicana, L. aethiopica.
- **Vector:** Phlebotomus sergenti, Phlebotomus salhi, Phlebotomus papatasi.
- **Clinical presentation:** Painless raised erythematous lesion with central ulcer and crust covering also known as 'Pizza based resembling ulcer'.
- **Treatment:** Antimony compound.

118. 57 years old man is admitted with primary complain of high grade fever of 104°C, along with malaise related symptoms for the last 4 days. Patient have had normal bowel movement with no complain of nausea or vomiting. Patient has a travel history to Uganda 2 months ago where he recalled have ulcerative lesion on his hand post fly bite at the same site. Patient is non smoker, non alcoholic with no known history of drug abuse. Patient is diabetic for the last 20 years and have been on metformin for the last 20 years and glifozins for the last 5 years. Patient is normotensive. On physical examination patient vitals were pulse rate 92 (probably due to high fever), Blood Pressure of 122/82, respiratory rate of 19 and fever of 103.8°C. Also there was presence of post cervical lymphadenopathy. Complete Blood Count analysis showed increased Eosinophils level.On giemsa staining following findings were observed.

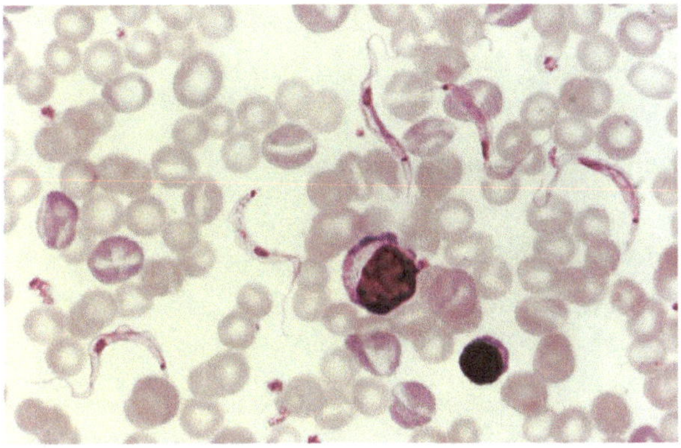

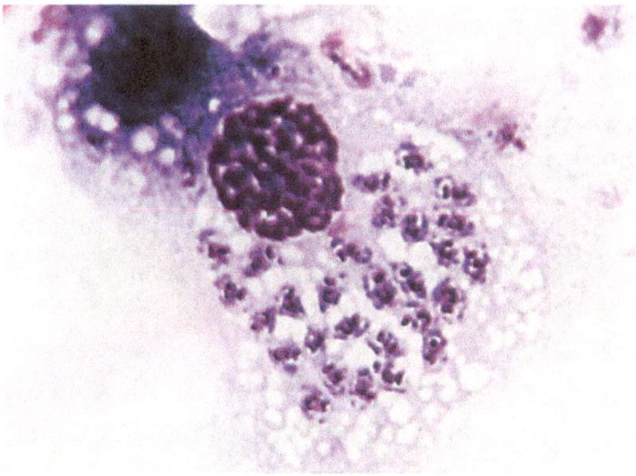

Which of the following is NOT correct regarding pathogenic organism?

A. Vector: Tsetse fly
B. Infective form is Metacyclic trypomastigote
C. Can lead on to neurological sequelae causing irritability, alteration of sleep cycle and personality disorder
D. Cultivation media: Weinmann media
E. Drug of choice: Praziquantel

Answer: E. Drug of choice is Praziquantel

Solution

- This is the case of sleeping sickness caused by Trypanosoma brucei.
- T. brucei Gambiense is known to cause West African sleeping sickness.
- T. brucei rhodesiense is known to cause East African sleeping sickness.
- **Vector:** Tsetse fly.
- **Infective form:** Metacyclic trypomastigote.

Clinical Features:

- Indurated painful chancre at site of tsetse fly bite.
- Hemolymphatic stage generally occurs weeks to months later of infection entering body.
  1. High grade fever.
  2. Post cervical lymphadenopathy – Winter bottom sign.
  3. Hepatosplenomegaly.
  4. Edema of hand and feet.
  5. Carditis may occur.
  6. Anemia.
- If not treated months to years later disease can enter neurological stage.
  1. Confusion.
  2. Irritability.
  3. Alteration of sleep pattern hence called sleeping sickness.

4. Personality disorder.

- Finally these symptoms can lead to coma and confirmed death.

Diagnosis:

- Under giemsa staining of blood or CSF we will observe trypomastigote.
- **Cultivation:** Weinmann media culture.
- **Serology:** Indirect Fluorescence antibody test, ELISA, NAAT.

Treatment:

- **T. brucei rhodesiense:**
  - o **Hemolymphatic stage:** Suramin.
  - o **Neurological stage:** Melarsoprol.
- **T. brucei Gambiense:**
  - o **Hemolymphatic stage:** Pentamidine.
  - o **Neurological stage:** Eflornithine.

119. 32 years old female was admitted to hospital with primary complain of abdominal pain in right hypochondrial region along with nausea and vomiting for the last 16 hours. Pain is continuous and sharp in nature. There is no associated diarrhea or abnormal bowel movement. There is no history of jaundice or hepatic disorder. On physical examination patient vitals were stable with Pulse rate of 73, Blood Pressure of 122/88, respiratory rate of 18 and normal temperature. There was no sign of icterus in the eye. On conducting Complete Blood Count analysis and LFT nothing abnormal was found. At this stage hepatic Ultrasound was done which showed presence of cyst with detached membrane or water Lilly sign or floating membrane sign. Which of the following is NOT correct regarding the pathogenic organism?

A. Definitive host for pathogenic organism is human

B. Pathogenic organism

C. First line management is PAIR

D. Accidental intermediate host are human

Answer: A. Definitive host for pathogenic organism is human

Solution

- This is the case of Hydatid cyst caused by Echinococcus granulosus.
- **Definitive host:** Dog.
- Man is the accidental intermediate host.
- **Organs affected:** Liver (most common) > lungs.

Symptoms and Signs:

1. Abdominal pain.
2. Nausea and vomiting.
3. Hepatomegaly.

Treatment:

- **Drug of Choice:** Albendazole.
- **Procedure of Choice:** PAIR (Percutaneous Aspiration Injection and Reaspiration).

120. 22 years old male comes with primary complain of watery diarrhea for the last 7 days. There is no presence of abdominal pain. There is no history of associated nausea or vomiting neither there is any presence of pus or blood on stool. There is no history of recent travel. But he did visited a restaurant 10 days ago to have beef and rice for dinner. Patient is non alcoholic, non smoker with no known history of drug abuse. Patient has been hypertensive for the last 10 years and have been on ACE inhibitor since then. On physical examination patient looks dull with no signs of dehydration. But his vitals are stable with Pulse rate of 78, Blood Pressure of 124/88, respiratory rate of 18 and his temperature was 99°C. There is no presence of icterus in the eye neither there is presence of any other sign of jaundice. His Complete Blood Count analysis showed increased Eosinophils and stools examination shows following presentation.

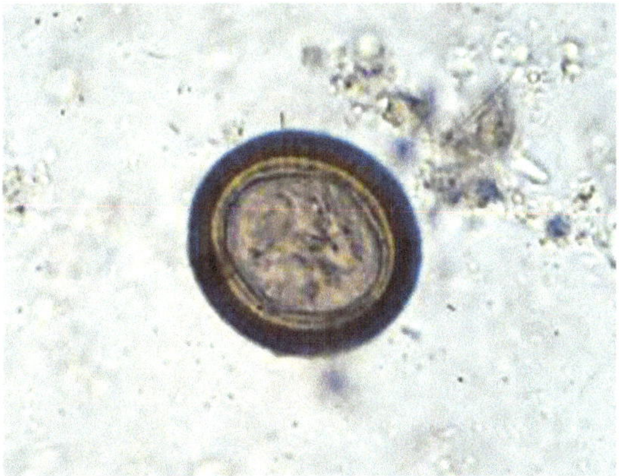

What is the infective form of pathogenic organism?

A. Cysticercus bovis
B. Rhabditiform larvae
C. Filariform larvae
D. Egg

Answer: A. Cysticercus bovis

Solution

- This is the case of infection caused by Taenia saginata.
- Taenia saginata comes under the classification of 'Cestodes'.
- **Definitive host:** Human's small intestine.
- **Infective form:** Cysticercus bovis.

Clinical Presentation:

1. Abdominal pain.
2. Diarrhea.
3. Anorexia.

Diagnosis:

- Stool test shows characteristic egg as shown below:

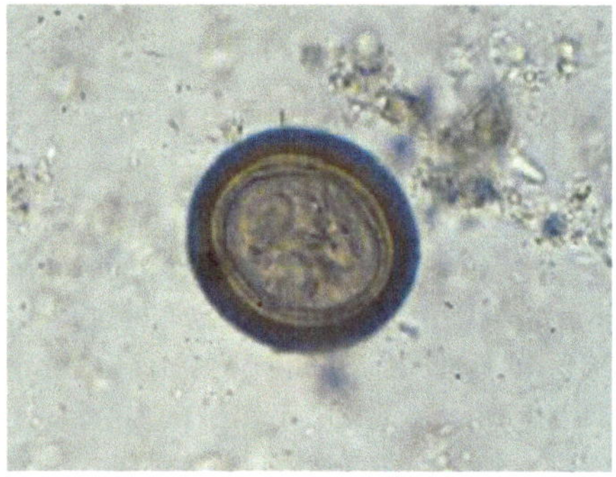

- **Treatment:** Niclosamide, praziquantel.

CHEAT BOOK FOR DRUG OF CHOICE

Organism	*Drug of Choice*
Salmonella	Ciprofloxacin
Proteus	Aminoglycosides and Cephalosporins
E. Coli	Cephalosporins, Fluoroquinolone, Trimethoprim-Sulfamethoxazole
Pseudomonas	Beta Lactams (Penicillin or Cephalosporins) + Aminoglycosides Carbapenem with Quinolones can be given in Conjunction with Aminoglycosides
Staphylococcus	First Line Penicillinase Penicillin like Oxacillin or Flucloxacillin + First or Second Generation Cephalosporins + Clindamycin or Quinolones
MRSA	Vancomycin or Daptomycin
Neisseria	Third Generation Cephalosporins
Streptococcus	Penicillin or Amoxicillin
Mycoplasma	First Choice Macrolide if not sensitive Fluoroquinolone and Tetra can be used
Clostridium	Ampicillin or Penicillin if not sensitive then give Clindamycin or Chloramphenicol Metronidazole can be given in combination with Ampicillin
Bacillus Anthracis	Ciprofloxacin, Doxyfloxacin, Levofloxacin
Coxiella Burnetti	Doxycycline + Hydroxychloroquine/Rifampicin/Ciprofloxacin for 2-4 years
Leptospira (Ictero Hemorrhagic Fever or Weil's)	**Mild:** Doxy, Ampicillin, Amoxicillin **Moderate/Severe:** Penicillin/Ceftoxime/Ceftriaxone/Doxycycline
Borrelia	Tetracycline/Macrolide
Listeria Monocytogenes	Ampicillin
Bordetella (Whooping Cough)	Macrolide
Nocardia	Cotrimoxazole, Linezolids, Cephalosporins
Brucella	Doxycyclin and Rifampin
Actinomyces	High Dose Penicillin
Nocardia	Cotrimoxazole Linezolids Cephalosporins
Haemophilus Influenzae	Third Generation Cephalosporins
Cryptosporidium	Nitazoxanide
Cyclospora and Cystoisospora	Cotrimoxazole
Malaria	Artemether-Lumefantrine or Atovaquone-Proguanil, Quinine and Mefloquine
Coxsackie	IVIG + Pleconaril

Contd.

Contd.

Influenza Virus	Oseltamivir, Zanamivir
Herpes	Acyclovir and Valacyclovir
CMV	Ganciclovir
Entamoeba Histolytica	Metronidazole + Poromomycin/Diloxanide
Naegleria Fowleri	Amphotericin B, Azithromycin, Fluconazole, Rifampin, Miltefosine and Dexamethasone
Candida	Azoles
Aspergillus	Voriconazole
Leishmania	Amphotericin B, Oral Miltefosine, Antimony Compound, Sitamaquine
Taenia	Nicolazamide, Praziquantel Neurocysticercosis: Albendazole, Praziquantel
Echinococcus Granulosus	Albendazole or Pair
Ancylostoma	Albendazole
Ascaris	Albendazole
Schistosoma	Praziquantel
Strongyloides Stercoralis	Ivermectin
Toxoplasma	Pyrimethamine + Folinic Acid + Clindamycin
Acute Chagas by Trypanosoma Cruzi	Nifurtimox or Benznidazole
Chronic Chagas by Trypanosoma Cruzi	Symptomatic treatment
Leishmania Tropica Lesion	Antimony compound
T. Brucei Rhodesiense	Hemolymphatic Stage: Suramin Neurological Stage: Melarsoprol
T. Brucei Gambiense	Hemolymphatic Stage: Pentamidine Neurological: Eflornithine